MAZEL TOV!

Originally published in Germany under the title
"Masel Tov – Die Moderne Jüdische Küche in aller Welt"
by Christian Verlag, in 2019.

Published in the United States in 2024
by Culina Cookbooks, an imprint of

Clevo Books
530 Euclid Ave #45
Cleveland, Oh 44115
www.clevobooks.com

Library of Congress Control Number: 2022947775
ISBN: 978-0-9973052-3-4
eBook ISBN: 978-1-68577-007-5

Printed in the USA

Translator: Michelle Standley
Editor: Cathryn Siegal-Bergman
English language layout: Ron Kretsch

First American Edition

MAZEL TOV!

MODERN JEWISH COOKING THROUGHOUT THE WORLD

RECIPES. PORTRAITS. STORIES.

BY LIV FLEISCHHACKER AND LUKAS GROSSMANN
PHOTOGRAPHY BY MARIA GROSSMANN AND MONIKE SCHUERLE
TRANSLATION BY MICHELLE STANDLEY

CONTENTS

PROLOGUE

Judaism has always played an important role in my family, even if it was more cultural than religious. In the 1930s, my paternal grandfather, Alfred Ginger Fleischhacker, was sent to England as part of what's known as the "children's transport" (Kindertransport), which saved him. Until the end of his life, he acted as a witness to the horrors of Nazi Germany and visited schools, travelling all over Germany to talk about his experiences.

Because of my grandfather, growing up I heard a lot about the Holocaust. When I was pretty young, my dad also insisted that I have six years of religious instruction. After that, though, I rebelled. I cut myself off from everything that had anything to do with Judaism. All my life, I'd been surrounded by it. At some point, I didn't want to hear about it anymore and simply couldn't.

Looking back, I see that I was being an arrogant teenager. I could afford to turn my back on my own family history: a luxury not available to everyone.

In my mid-twenties, I found my way back. As a journalist, I had gotten pretty involved in writing about culinary and drinking culture. That led me to getting increasingly interested in subjects related to Jewish culinary culture and I ended up sorting of stumbling my way back home. When it came to my family's history, I found it easier to connect through subjects that were meaningful to me and with which I felt comfortable. I wrote about Jewish food culture and the history of food in my hometown, Berlin. These days, I'm engaged with Judaism in some form or another nearly every day, mostly from the angle of its cuisine.

Several years later, in the summer of 2016, my friend Laurel Kratochvila, who runs Fine Bagels in Berlin, asked me if I would like to organize a Jewish food festival with her. We both had the feeling that the time was ripe. A lot of Jewish food culture has been lost. More recently, though, there has been a slow but steady re-emergence of it in the German capital. Laurel and I were both sure that it only needed a platform to give it a bit more attention. In March 2017, "Nosh Berlin" took place. A week filled with workshops, panel discussions, readings, film screenings, markets, and of course, an incredible amount of food. We considered it a huge success!

In early 2017, Sonya Mayer from Christian Verlag got in touch with me. The photographer, Maria Grossmann, had proposed making a book like this one, and Sonya wanted to make it happen. After discussing it, we agreed that we wanted to present the diversity of Jewish cooking. It's incredibly multifaceted and hasn't received all that much attention in Germany.

We all agreed: Jewish cuisine is a world cuisine, there is no one "definitive" version. Some foods, like matzo and cholent, are closely tied to Jewish tradition and dietary commandments. Even if there are regional differences in how they are interpreted, their core remains the same. In general, you might say that Jewish food is more of a cultural movement in which everyone can participate as much or as little as they want to.

With *Mazel Tov!* we try to represent as many cultures as possible. From Israeli-Moroccan meatballs to gefilte fish, from Mexican jalapeño-matzto-ball soup to Danish raisin crowns, from noodle kugel to bagels and Yugoslav chestnut bars. Jewish food is as colorful as the people of Jewish descent. They come from everywhere and the food represents that. From throughout the diaspora, the wandering Jews brought their traditions with them to their new homes. They adapted their cooking practices to these new settings but also found inspiration from them as well.

Many people who think of Jewish food often imagine Eastern European food and certain traditional Sabbat dishes. Of course, that's not entirely inaccurate. Eastern European culinary culture is an essential part of Ashkenazi cooking. And traditional Sabbat dishes, cooked overnight, can be found in many Jewish subcultures. But there is so much more! Jewish cooking is a lot more varied than people realize. A lot of it's kosher but a lot of it isn't. To take but one example, in Israel most people share a love for regional, fresh cooking that takes inspiration from other cultures in the Middle East. People nonetheless have a lot of different ideas about what constitutes Jewish cuisine and culture. Some Israelis observe kosher laws, some don't. Those who don't may choose not to simply because they want to enjoy the variety of different types of seafood that are available, including things like shellfish, which are not permitted according to kosher laws.

Our recipes are Ashkenazi and Sephardic in origin, modern and traditional, and have one eye on the past and another on the future. The recipes are not kosher. We decided against the religious connection because we wanted to focus on the diversity of Jewish cuisine and kosher recipes play no part in non-kosher kitchens. If you want to cook kosher, you have to follow many rules, not the least of which is remembering to use properly cleaned utensils and pans.

Our contributors generously dug into their family treasure troves to share their recipes, and for that I can't thank them enough. I'd also like to thank them for sharing their stories with us so openly and honestly.

The selection of contributors came about organically. Everyone who participated in the book suggested other people and that's how we ended up with our 19 contributors. I know many of them personally and find their stories and thoughts about Jewish cuisine interesting. Although not all of them are professional chefs, a good part of them works in some

way with food. Some are gifted amateur chefs. All share an interest in Jewish cuisine and how it connects us globally.

The main aim of this book is to present the range of Jewish cuisine and perhaps to broaden horizons a bit when it comes to Jewish food. But I'm also interested in the stories that emerged through organizing this book: they are stories that were passed on in families and thus live on orally. Hopefully, in the written form, they will also find readers in the future. My greatest desire is to bring you a little bit of Jewish cuisine and possibly introduce you to something new to add to your own collection of family recipes. Mazel tov!

—Liv Fleischhacker

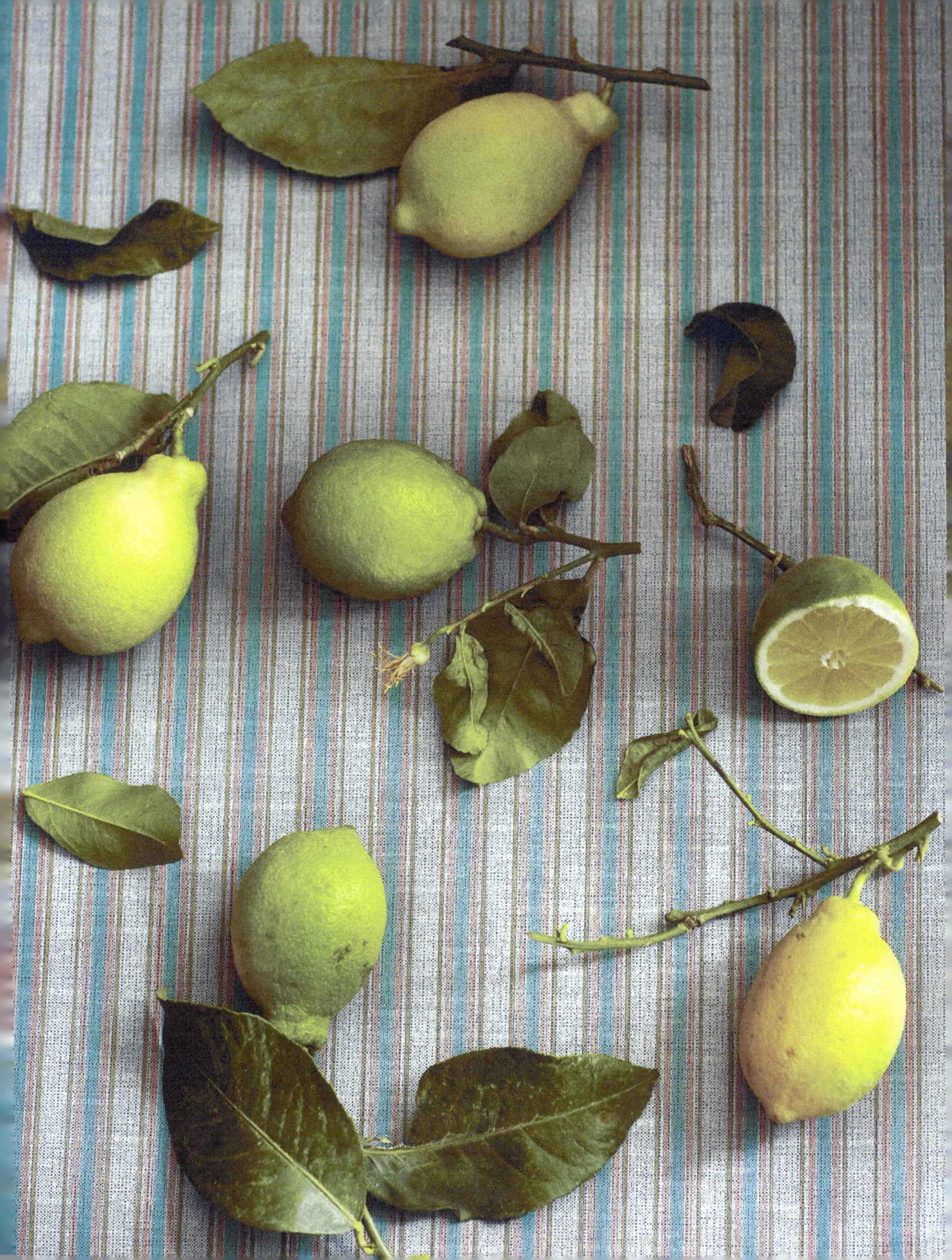

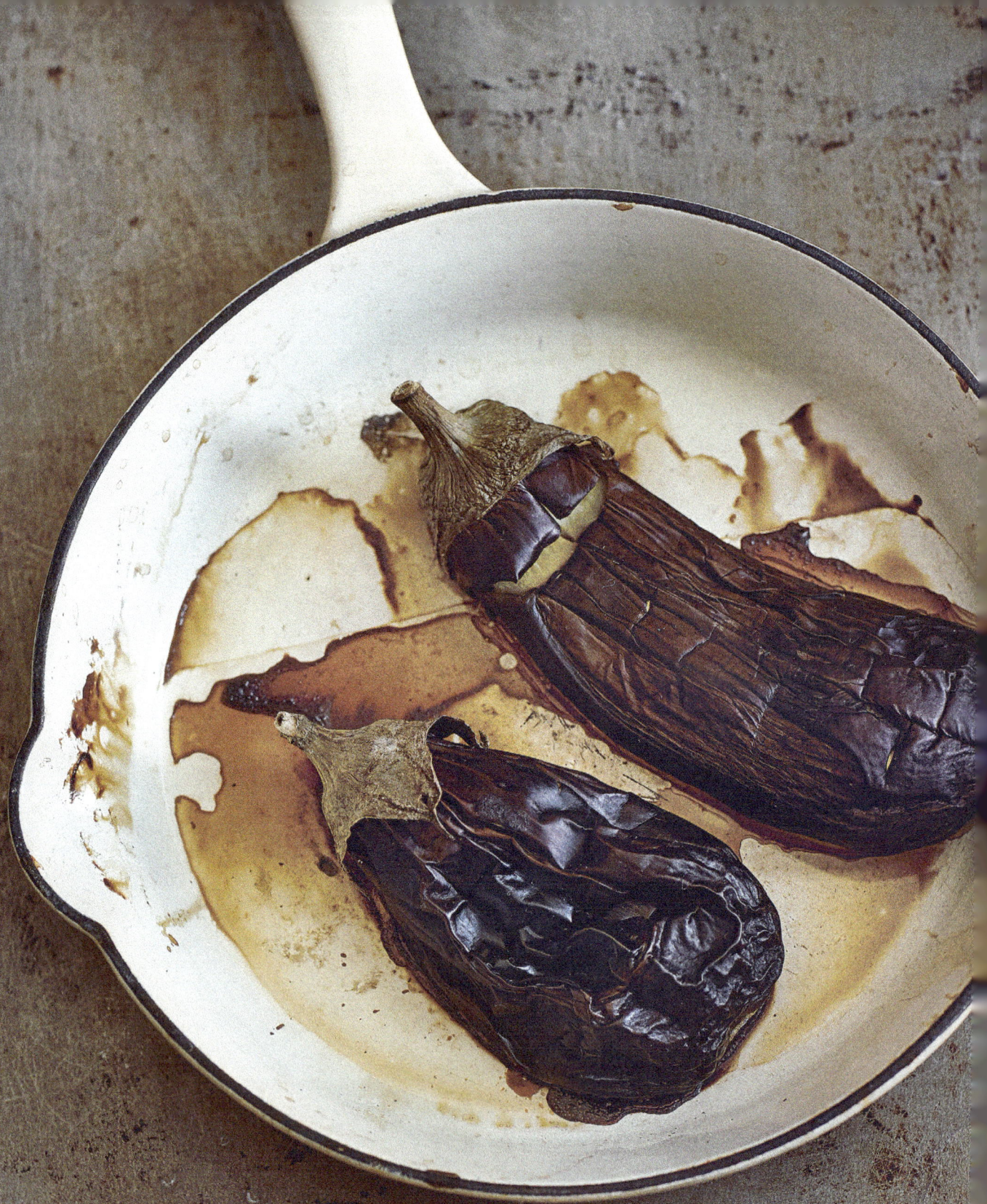

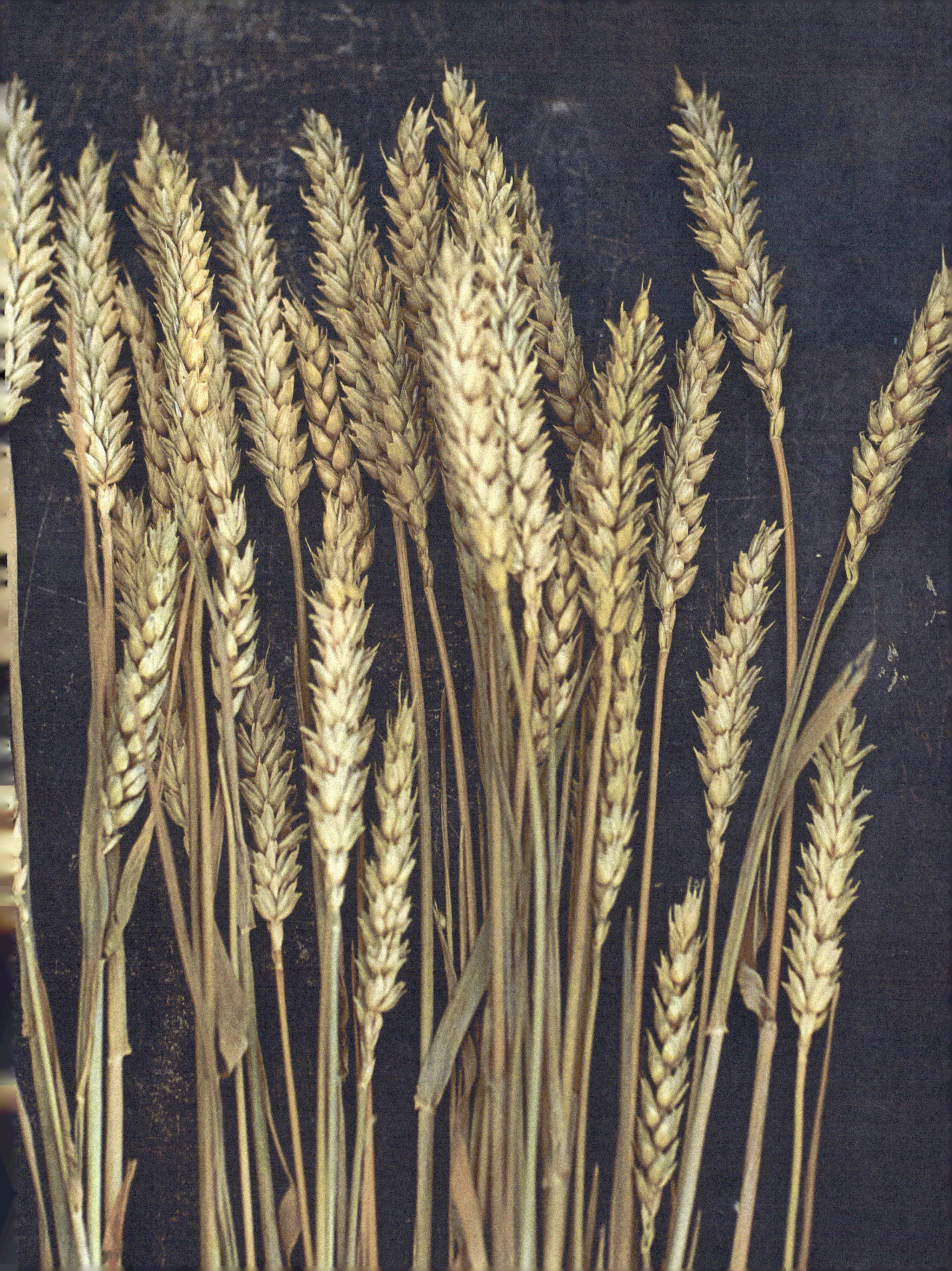

GIL HOVAV,
Tel Aviv

EVERY DISH
TELLS A STORY

With his warm and kind manner, Gil Hovav is the quintessential host. He is also a living legend of Israeli cuisine. Gil began his career as a restaurant critic; has been a part of the creation, production, and hosting of a number of Israel's most popular television shows; and has written more than 15 cookbooks and three novels. His work on Israeli cuisine has played a major part in making it as popular as it is today.

Born in Jerusalem in 1962, Gil grew up in a large household. His family lived with his maternal grandmother, who was in charge of the kitchen. He loved the Sephardic food that she cooked for the family. His parents had important positions at the Israeli Broadcasting Authority, which meant that the family often ate out. That was pretty unusual in Israel in the 1960s and 1970s. It was almost considered indecent. Such an upbringing, though, allowed Gil to experience a full range of restaurants and provided him with a sort of training to later become a restaurant critic.

Gil maintains that when it comes to food, "There is no ultimate truth. What tastes good to me, the person next to me might not like. To write about it, you have to make comparisons between different types of food and dishes." Gil got into writing by chance: As a student, he cleaned houses, taught Arabic, and worked as a bartender. To pay tuition, he started looking for a fourth job. He called his local newspaper and said to the editor, "I want to write." He started by writing about bars and that launched his career as a bar critic. He worked as deputy editor-in-chief at almost every newspaper in Israel. That's how he got into television. These days television is so saturated with food that Gil has chosen to focus on history and travel.

His fascination with food started early on. His grandmother would make kubaneh bread for every Sabbat brunch. He would fight with his siblings over who got the crispiest pieces. He didn't learn to cook from his grandmother, however. That's because

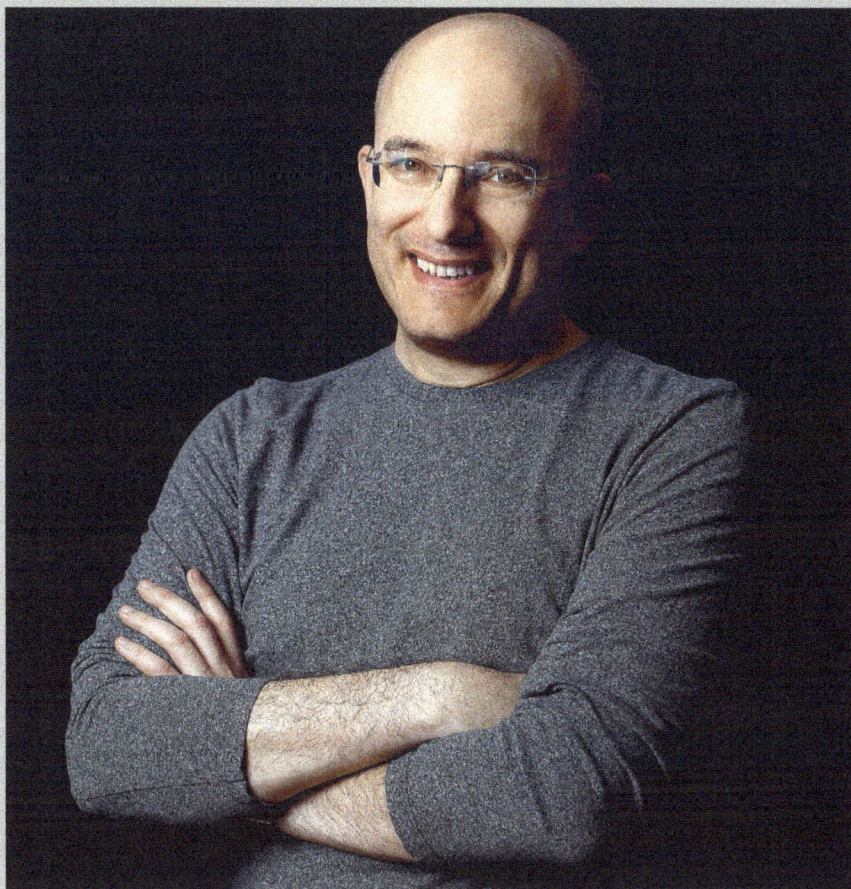

Gil Hovav started his career as a restaurant critic. Today he is a successful author, recipe developer, and chef.

traditionally Sephardic men weren't allowed in the kitchen; people said they brought only dirt and bad luck. On the day that she died, Gil was a 20-year-old soldier and began cooking to remember her. Such an act was an expression of his belief that cooking is closely tied to storytelling, "Taste and memory are very closely linked. Every dish tells a story."

As a restaurant critic, Gil has to eat out ten times a week. However, he loves to cook and is always happy to come home after a long week of travel and make something for himself. He's not into elaborate, fancy dishes. He loves simple things that remind him of his family and his home. Laughing, Gil describes his approach to cooking as something akin to that of an elderly aunt. When he's been on the road for a long time, the first dish that he makes at home is a big plate of fresh vegetables, served with a little olive oil and salt. It's accompanied by a piece of Israeli bread and olives, "For me, that's the taste of Israel, fresh and

local." Gil also likes to eat hot and spicy carrot salad. Instead of relying on the beet's natural sweetness, he seasons them generously with lemon, olive oil, spring onions, and hot peppers. The longer the salad can steep, the better. After two days, it tastes incredible. A fresh dish that will brighten any table.

When he wants comfort food, Gil cooks his paternal grandmother's kubaneh bread. The bread is meant for brunch on Sabbat. When he was a kid, his grandmother used to prepare it for the family every Saturday. Traditionally, it's baked overnight and is eaten in the morning. Because the bread is in the oven for so long, it develops a special flavor. The individual rolls are smeared with butter before going in the oven. They thus caramelize slowly: without any sugar! Gil bakes kubaneh with a proportional wheat/rye mixture, making it a little healthier. You can replace half of the butter with olive oil, if you want. The kubaneh is served with butter and zhug: a spicy Yemeni sauce flavored with

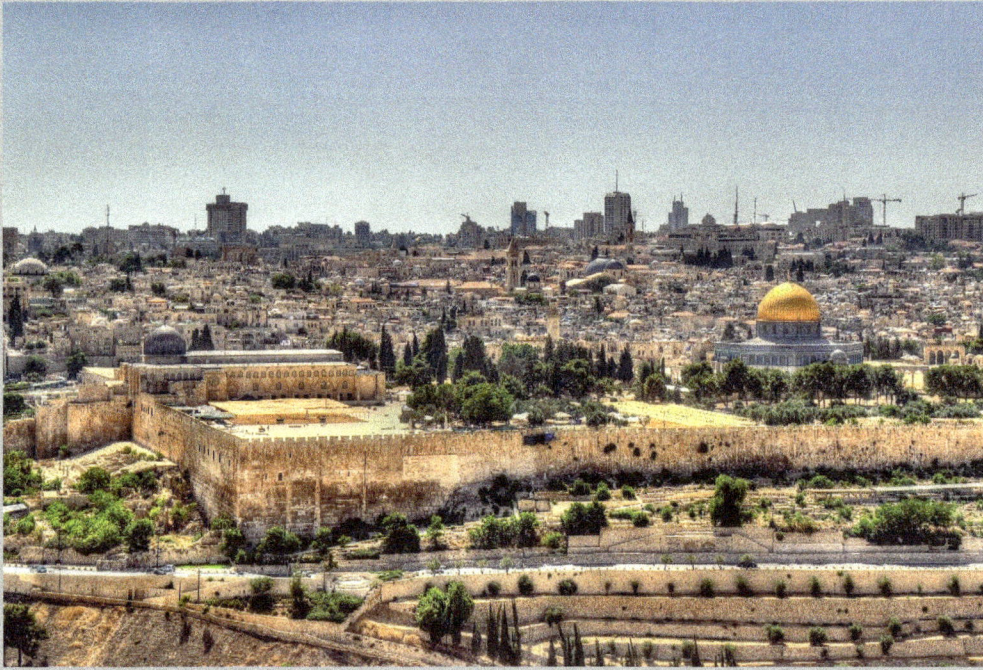

Photos to the left and to the right: Jerusalem, where Gil Hovav was born.

cilantro and coriander seeds and, in which cardamom, cumin, parsley, and lots of chili play a leading role. Served with the buttery rolls, zhug has an invigorating effect; it gives even the biggest morning grouch a bit of pleasure at the Saturday morning breakfast table. Cream cheese and jam go well with kubaneh as do freshly sliced tomatoes tossed with good olive oil and salt or even a fried egg. What's most important for Gil is that zhug is always on hand. A Yemeni proverb says, "When kubaneh is on the table, all other breads must bow." It's a very, very special dish and Gil tries to bake it himself every Saturday to remember his grandmother and to remind him of the smell of home.

Gil travels frequently all across the globe and opens up Yemeni pop-up restaurants. Because his grandmother was very poor, it fills Gil with pride when he makes her kubaneh bread for people and they say that they love it. Every time this happens, he thinks to himself: "This is for you, Grandma."

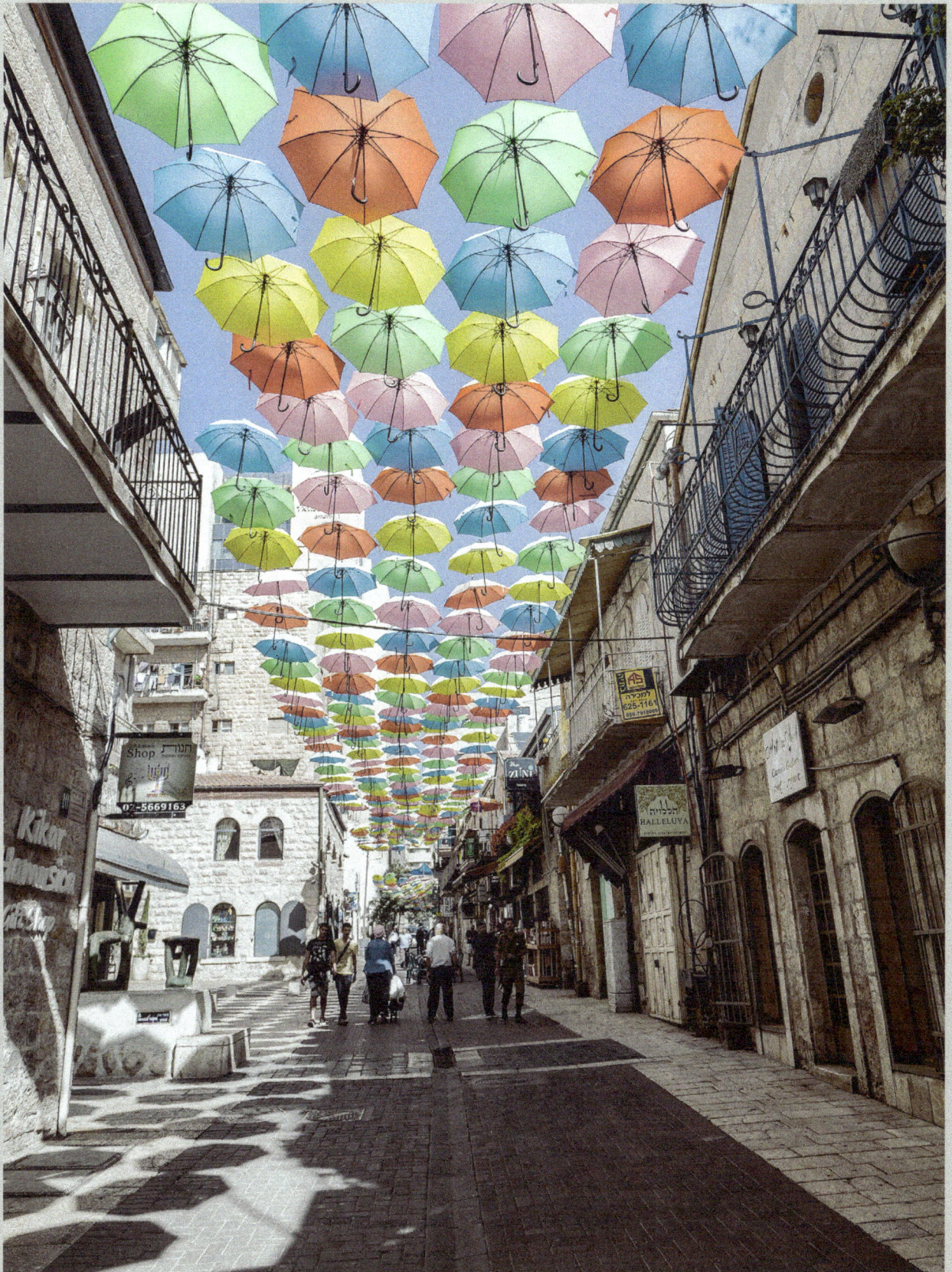

KUBANEH —YEMMENI SABBAT BREAD

SERVES 6 / MAKES 1 LOAF

PREPARATION: 40 MIN.
RISING TIME: 90 MIN.
BAKING TIME: 60 MIN.

DOUGH
4 cups (500 g) all-purpose
    flour
½ cup (60 g) whole wheat flour
2 ¼ teaspoons (7 g) or 1
    envelope active dry yeast
1 tablespoon sugar
3 teaspoons salt
2 cups (480 mL) lukewarm
    water

FINAL STEPS
All-purpose flour for work
    surface
11 tablespoons (150 g) butter

DOUGH

Knead the flours, yeast, sugar, salt, and water in a bowl until a slightly sticky dough is formed. Cover the dough and let rise in a warm and dark place for 45 minutes.

FINAL STEPS

1. Transfer the dough to a lightly floured work surface and knead with your hands for 2 minutes until a smooth dough is formed.
2. Divide the dough into 10 equal portions. On a lightly floured work surface, turn each portion of dough into balls with the hollow of your hand. Working in a circular motion and with gentle pressure, work until the top of the ball is closed and slightly taut. Place the balls on a baking sheet, cover with a cloth and let rise for 15 minutes.

3. Meanwhile, melt the butter in a saucepan

4. One at a time, grease each piece of dough with a little melted butter, spreading it all over. On a clean work surface, roll into a thin rectangle, measuring about 6 x 8 inches. Then brush again with melted butter. Fold the dough in half from the longer side to form a narrow rectangle. Then roll it up into a cylinder. Prepare 10 dough rosettes in this way.

5. Grease a 9-inch springform baking pan with butter and stack the rosettes in it. Cover with a cloth and let rise for 30 minutes.

6. Preheat the oven to 350°F.

7. Bake for 60 minutes. (Note: If the bread turns too brown early, simply cover the surface with a layer of aluminum foil)..

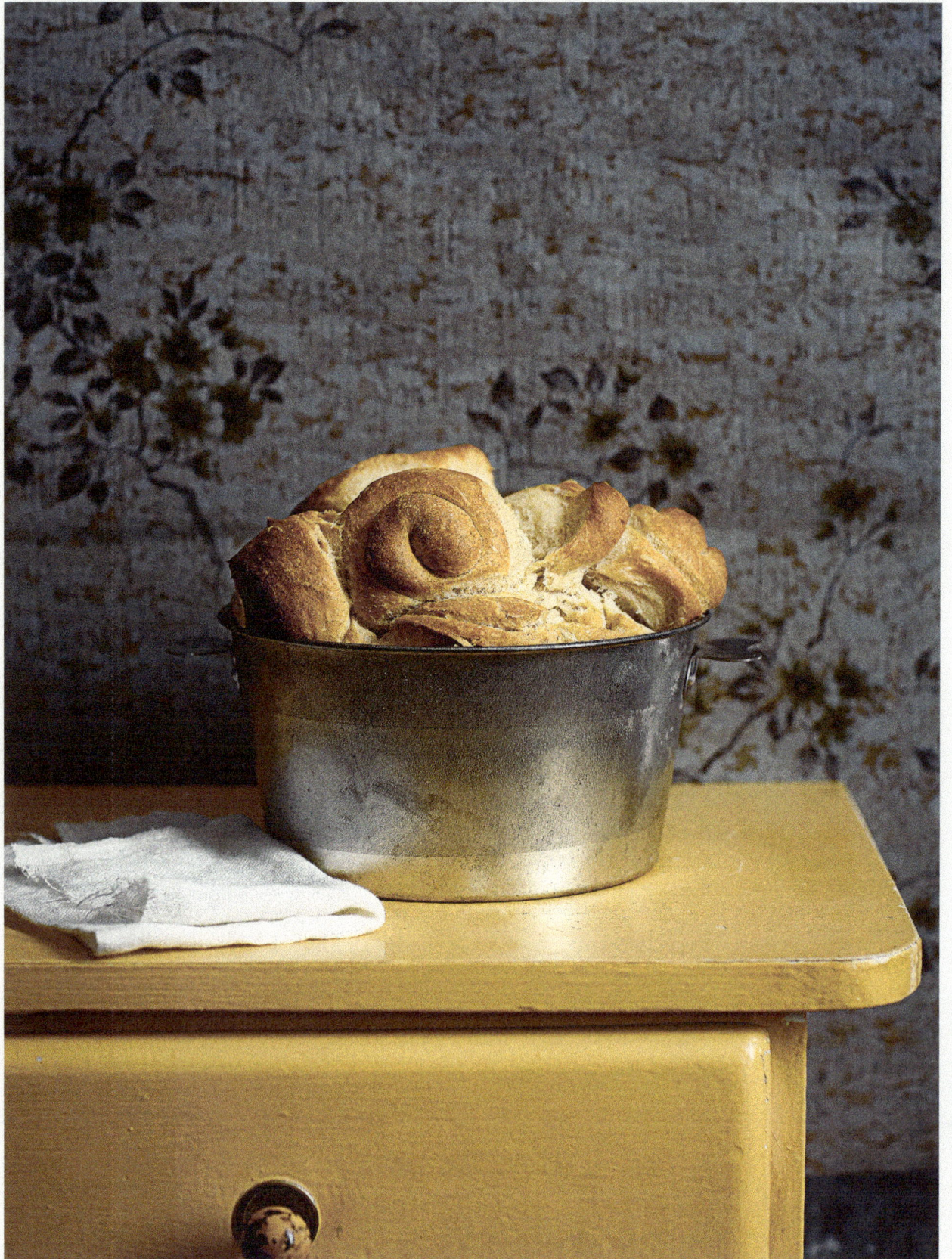

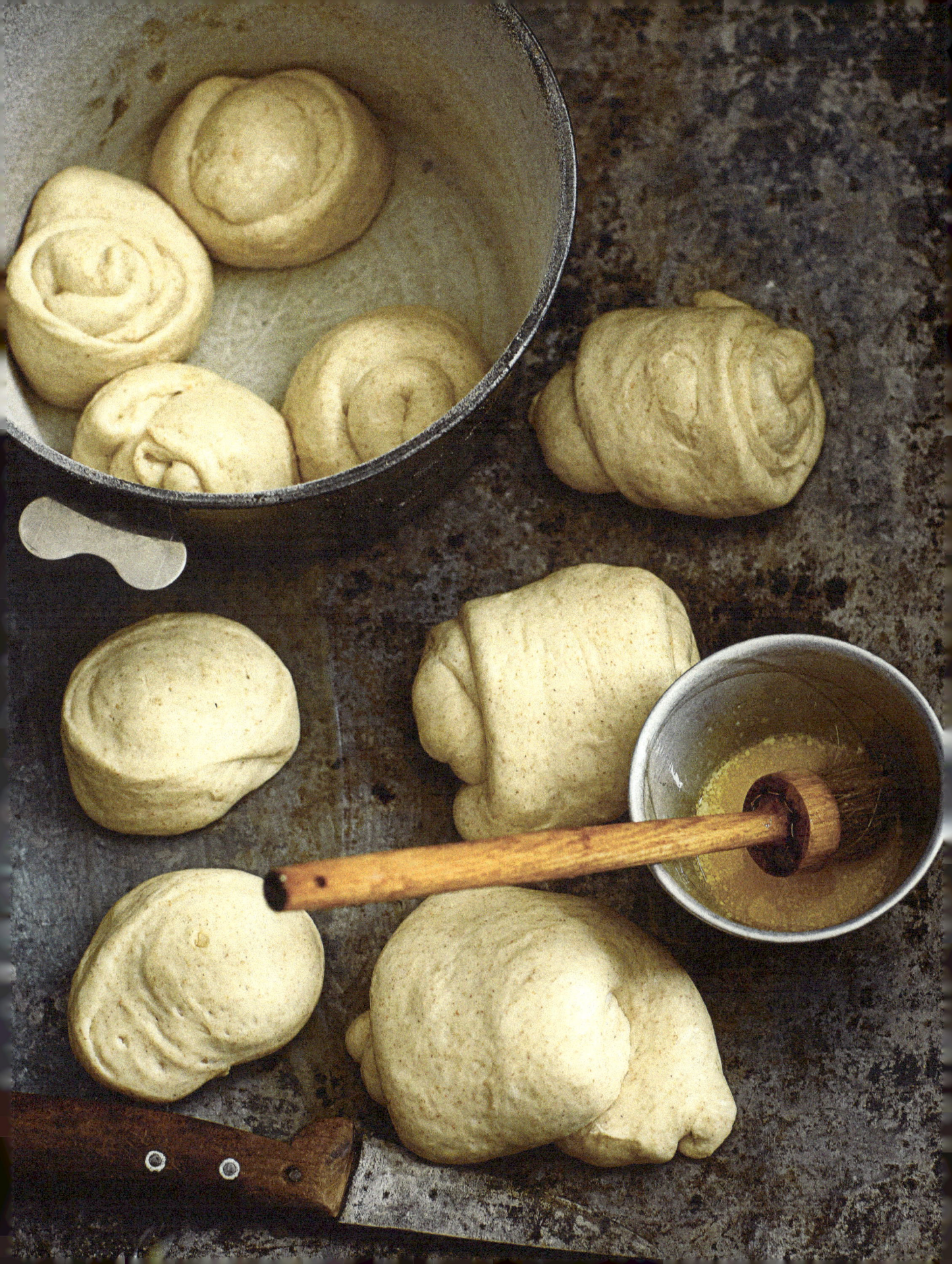

ZHUG
—YEMMENI SPICY SALSA

MAKES ABOUT 1 JAR
  (1 ½ cups)
PREPARATION: 15 MIN.

ZHUG
½ bulb garlic
8 fresh hot green chilies
  (such as jalapeños)
1 bunch cilantro
½ tablespoon black
  peppercorns
½ tablespoon coriander
  seeds
½ tablespoon cardamom
  seeds
½ tablespoon cumin seeds
½ tablespoon salt
3 tablespoons olive oil

ZHUG

1. Peel the garlic, remove the stems from the chili peppers, and blend to a coarse paste in a food processor.
2. Wash the cilantro, shake dry, coarsely chop, and add to the chili paste in the food processor.
3. Crush the peppercorns, coriander seeds, caraway seeds, and salt in a mortar and add to the chili paste in the food processor along with the oil. Blend until you get a fine, bright green paste.
4. Pour the zhug into a jar, seal tightly and store in the refrigerator for a maximum of 8 weeks.

Tip: The paste is very spicy and should be used judiciously. It tastes great with pastrami, pulled beef or even shakshuka.

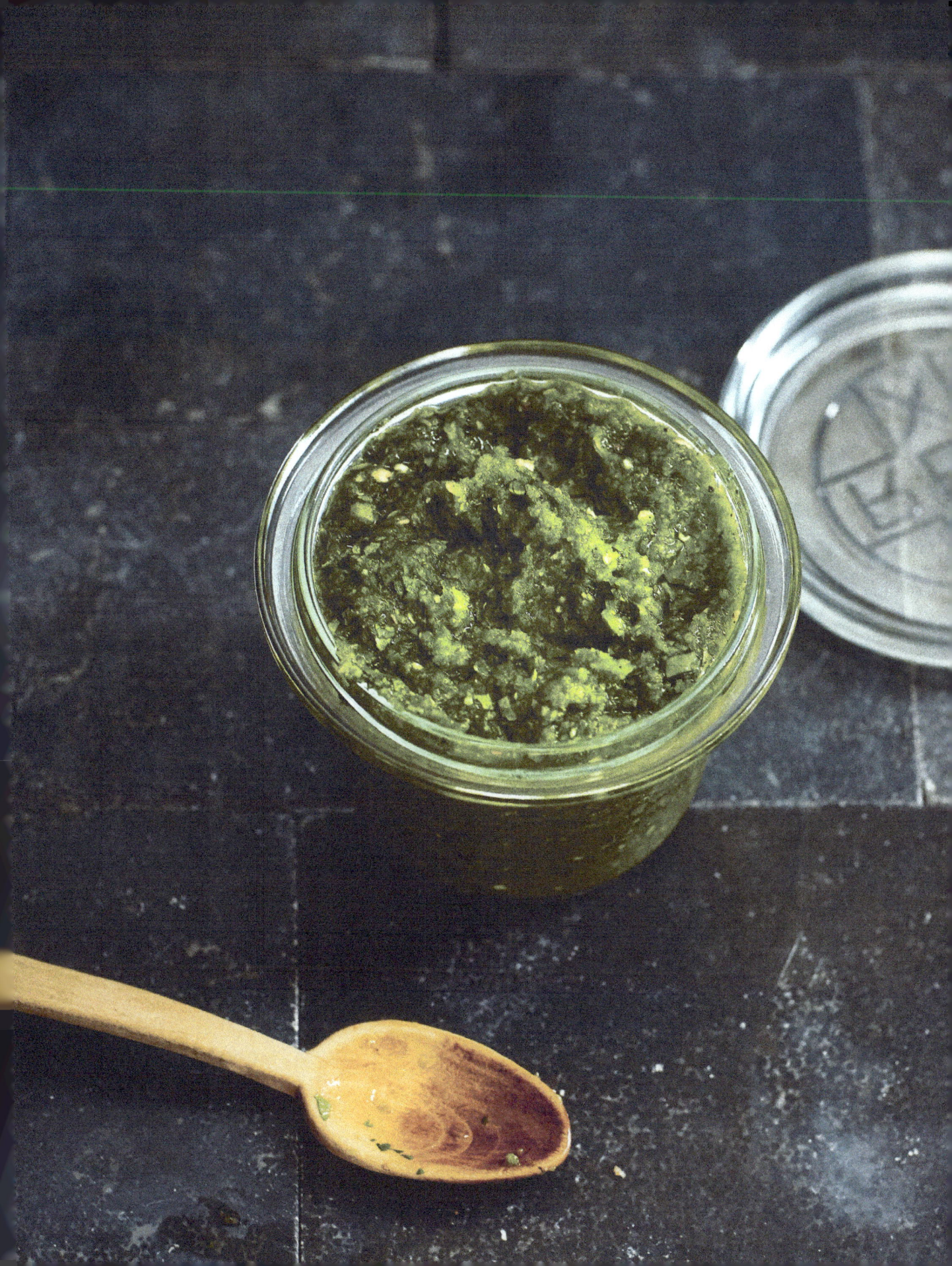

SPICY ISRAELI CARROT SALAD

SERVES 4
PREPARATION: 20 MIN.

CARROT SALAD
2 organic lemons
6 large carrots
1 bunch of cilantro
2 spring onions
1 hot green chili pepper
   (such as jalapeño)
3 cloves of garlic
Salt
Freshly ground black
   pepper
1 pinch of sugar
3-4 tablespoons olive oil

CARROT SALAD

1. Wash the lemons thoroughly. Squeeze the juice into a large bowl. Chop 1 squeezed lemon very finely and add to the bowl. Thoroughly wash and peel the carrots and finely slice with a slicer or knife.

2. Wash the cilantro and thoroughly pat dry. Finely chop the stems and coarsely chop the leaves. Clean the spring onions and cut into fine rings. Halve the chili pepper, remove the seeds, and cut into thin strips. Mince the garlic.

3. Mix everything in the bowl. Season the salad with salt, freshly ground pepper, and 1 pinch of sugar and let it sit for a few minutes. Finally, mix in the olive oil and serve in a bowl.

Tip: The salad goes well with hearty lamb or beef stews. It's also good alongside other side dishes, like hummus.

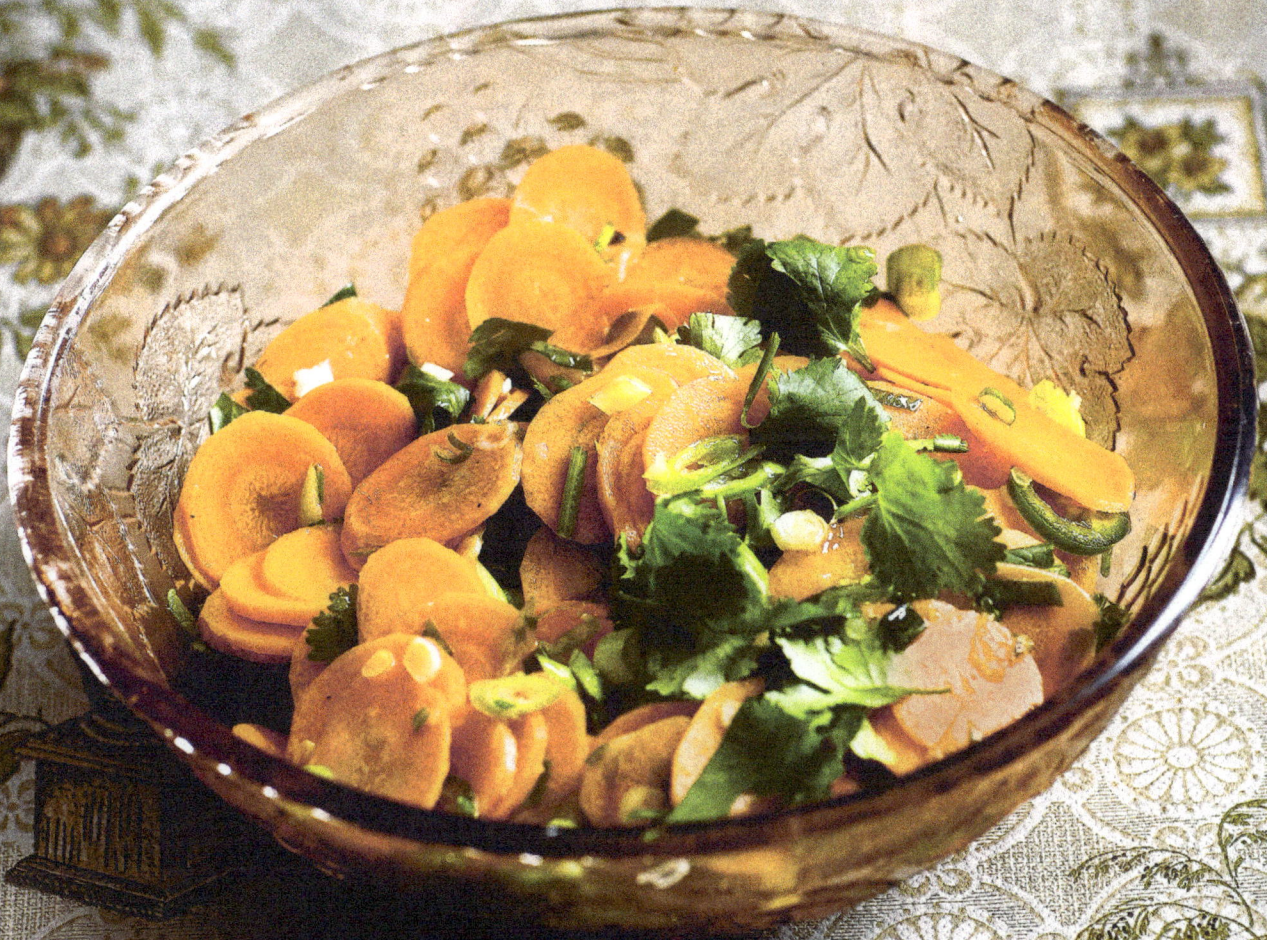

MATAN CHOUFAN,
Tel Aviv

FOOD
FOR SHARING

When he was young, Matan Choufan refused to eat a lot of things: onions, tomatoes, eggplants. In fact, he didn't like to eat almost anything related to the food where he grew up, Israel. But the older he got, the more he ventured. When he joined the army, he started eating avocados and eggplants. But the big change took place when he later moved out of his parents' house in Ilad, in the south of Israel, to Tel Aviv, about five hours away. In Tel Aviv he started cooking for himself—because he had to! On Friday nights, he cooked for Sabbat with friends from Ilad. It started out simple: meatballs in red sauce. With each successive week, though, he became more ambitious and dared to use more complex ingredients.

He may have started out as a somewhat picky eater, but he quickly made up for lost time and took up writing about food. He started while still in the army and then continued to write about it when he was in college. But,

initially at least, he didn't pursue food writing as a career. Instead, after the army, he studied communications and later got a job as a communications manager. But he continued to write about food on the side for various publications, eventually including such major publications as Haaretz, Israel's oldest newspaper. When he was 25, he also started a blog, inspired by his parents' Tunisian roots, "The Tunisian Table." It started out pretty basic, as a place to record notes related to cooking. Over time, it grew into something more ambitious. He used it to preserve his family's history, through their recipes; to share new ones that he had discovered or was testing out; and to feature guest entries as well. Finally, after years of working in communications and only writing about food on the side, he decided that his true passion was food. He quit his full-time job and devoted himself to working as a writer, branding consultant, and editor for topics related to food. Today he's the director of content at

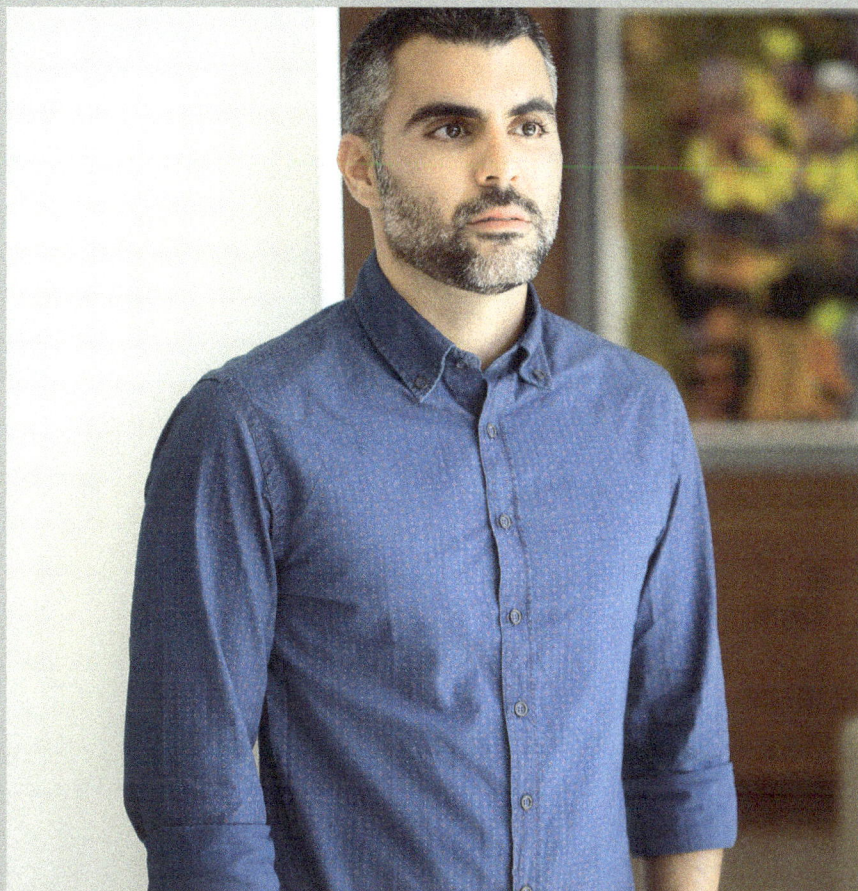

A writer, editor, and consultant who writes about food for the Israeli newspaper *Haaretz*, Matan Choufan lovingly cooks his way through his grandmother's recipes.

a culinary institute in Tel Aviv, devoted to promoting local food culture.

Matan's approach to cooking is strongly influenced by his mother and his two grandmothers. Many of his recipes come from his paternal grandmother. His parents are happy when he publishes one of her recipes and stories in Haaretz. Through his work, he does a lot of research and always learns something new about his own family history and Tunisian cooking. He's explored, for instance, the close connection between cooking in Tunisia and southern Italy. Their physical proximity and the large amount of migration between the countries has meant a constant exchange between their two cooking cultures. This exchange has influenced the cooking in his family and thus Matan's cooking too. His grandmother, who lived in Tunis, had a lot of Italian neighbors and learned many recipes from them. She was always happy to share her stories

and recipes with him. She lived to be nearly 100 years old and was still active and healthy even to the end of her long life. Matan is quite sure that no one cooks as well as she did. He still uses her recipes at home; for Sabbat he likes to cook her couscous, her soups, and her meatballs, all served, with Tunisian salads.

Matan's married now and doesn't return home for every holiday. He celebrates with his own family at his home in Tel Aviv. For Sukkot, he still prepares his grandmother's fish cakes. This is important because his partner's family cooks a lot of Ashkenazi food, and he always likes to bring something of himself, of his tradition, to the table.

Matan's food is full of flavor, often very spicy, and colorful. Lots of olive oil, lots of garlic, lots of spice! Food for sharing. That's how he celebrates his grandmother and his ancestors in his work and in his daily life.

TUNISIAN FISH FOR SHABBAT

SERVES 4
PREPARATION: 45 MIN.

BELL PEPPER SAUCE
4 red bell peppers
4 cloves of garlic
2 tablespoons vegetable
  oil
1 teaspoon cumin seeds
1 teaspoon harissa (North
  African spice blend)
1 teaspoon sweet paprika
Salt

FISH
1 ¾ lb (800 g) cod fillet,
  skin removed
½ lemon
Salt

TO SERVE
Some fresh cilantro,
  leaves only
Freshly grilled challah

BELL PEPPER SAUCE
1. Wash the peppers, cut them in half, and remove the stems, seeds, and white membranes. Chop into big chunks. Coarsely chop the garlic cloves. Purée the peppers and garlic in a food processor.
2. Heat the vegetable oil in a wide, shallow saucepan or skillet over medium-high heat. Add the cumin seeds and toast until fragrant. Add the pepper-garlic purée, harissa spice mix, and paprika, and bring to a boil. Reduce the heat and simmer with a lid on top for about 20 minutes. Season with salt to taste.

FISH
If necessary, remove any bones from the cod fillet, wash under running water and thoroughly pat dry. Cut the fish into bite-sized pieces about ¾-inch thick. Place the fish pieces in a pot, side by side, add the sauce, sprinkle with a squeeze of lemon and season with a pinch of salt. Put a lid on top and cook for about 10-15 minutes at low heat.

TO SERVE
Garnish with cilantro and serve with challah.

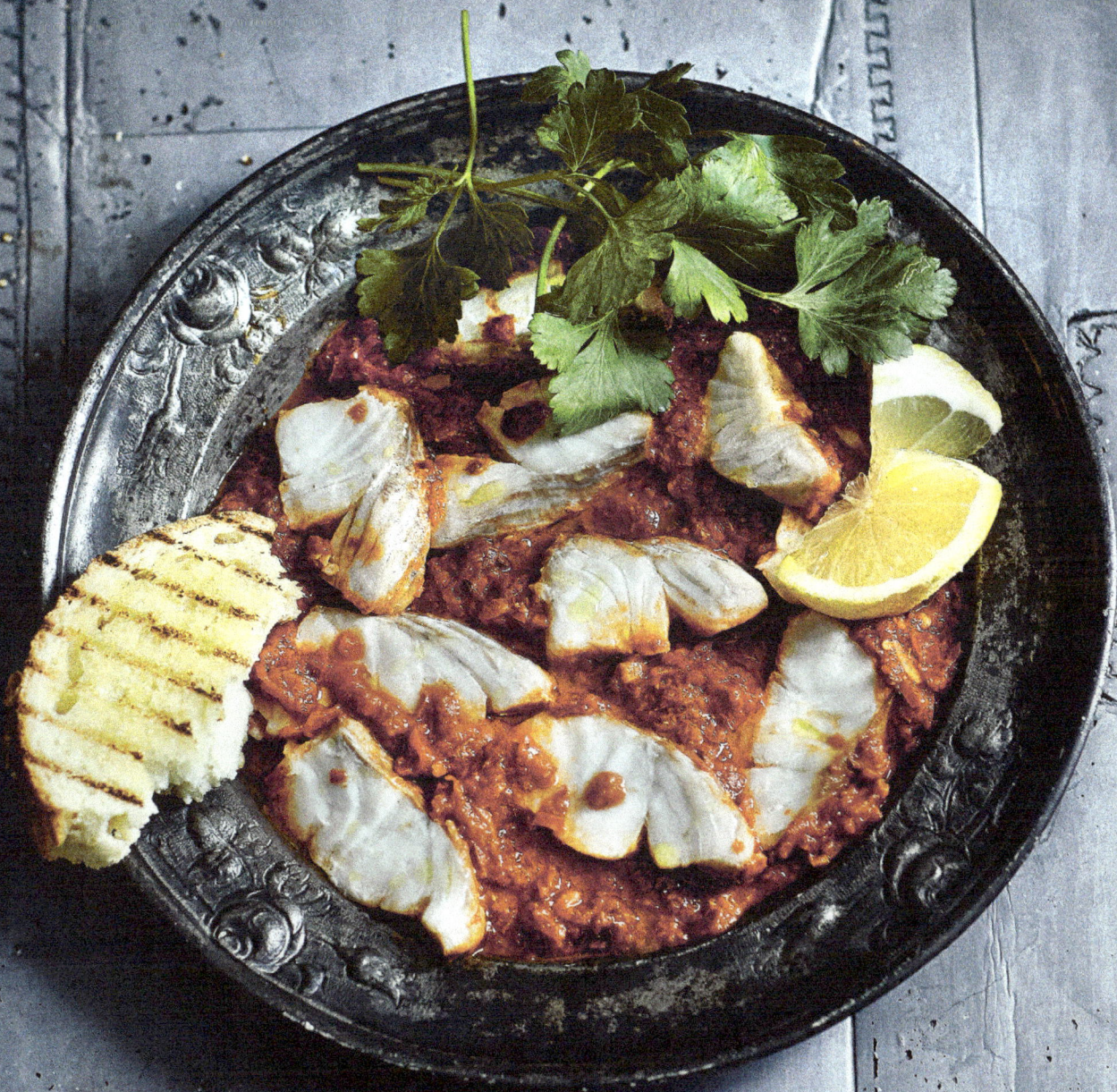

ITALIAN KREPLACH WITH BEANS AND BOTTARGA

SERVES 4
PREPARATION: 60 MIN.
SOAKING, RESTING &
COOKING TIME: 34 HRS.

BEAN FILLING
2 cups (220 g) dried white
    beans
2 cups (500 mL) olive oil
1 garlic bulb
5 sprigs of thyme
1 bay leaf salt
Freshly ground black
    pepper

DOUGH
¾ cup (165 g) fine durum
    wheat flour (semola di
    grano duro)
1 1/3 cups (165 g) all-
    purpose flour
1 garlic bulb confit (see
    "bean filling" above)
3 eggs

BEAN FILLING

1. Put the dried beans in a pot, cover with about 10 cups of cold water, soak for 24 hours, changing the water twice. Drain and rinse, then put back in the pot with about 6 cups of water. Boil for 1 hour and drain.

2. Preheat the oven to 210°F. Heat the olive oil in an ovenproof pot to 210°F. Add the cooked beans, the whole garlic bulb, the thyme sprigs, the bay leaf, and a pinch each of salt and pepper. Place the pot in the oven and cook for 8 hours.

3. Remove the garlic bulb and set aside to prepare the dough. Remove the herbs and drain the beans. (Note: the oil is no longer needed but can be used later). Using a potato masher, mash the beans into a fine paste and season with salt and freshly ground pepper.

DOUGH

In a bowl, mix the flours, then on a lightly floured work surface form into a mound, make a well in the middle. Remove the skins from the soft garlic cloves and, in a small bowl mash into a fine paste. Put the paste and the eggs into the well in the flour. Using your hands, mix the flour with the eggs and garlic, moving from the outside in, and knead into a smooth dough. If it is too sticky, add more flour. Cover in plastic wrap and let rest in the refrigerator for 1 hour.

FINAL STEPS

Some fine durum wheat
  semolina (semola di
  grano duro) for work
  surface
1 egg
Salt
1 shallot
2 tablespoons (30 g)
  butter
2 tablespoons olive oil

TO SERVE

1 oz (25 g) bottarga (salted
  mullet roe

FINAL STEPS

1. After it has rested, use a pasta machine to roll out the
dough into thin sheets. Start at the highest level and roll
out in several passes to the second, thinnest level; this
makes the dough elastic and easier to shape without tearing.
After each pass through the machine, sprinkle the sheets
of dough with a little durum wheat semolina. Alternatively,
you can roll out the dough by hand into thin sheets, about
1/8-inch thick. From the sheets of dough, cut out circles with
a diameter of about 3 inches. Place 1 heaping teaspoon of
bean filling in the center and brush the edges with a little
beaten egg. Fold the circles into a crescent shape and brush
the pointed ends with a little egg as well. Then press them
together to make the typical tortellini shape.

2. Bring plenty of water to the boil in a large saucepan,
salt generously and cook the tortellini in it for 6-8
minutes until they rise to the surface.

3. While the tortellini cooks, peel the shallot and julienne,
i.e., cut it into thin strips. In a large skillet, over medium-
high heat, add the butter, whisking it continuously as it
melts so that it reaches a frothy state and until the whey,
or the top white layer of the butter as it separates, is
golden brown. Add the olive oil and shallot and sweat
them for 2 minutes until translucent. Remove the cooked
tortellini from the pot, scooping them out of the water
with a slotted spoon. Add them to the skillet, dripping
wet. Sauté until the sauce is emulsified and shiny.

TO SERVE

Divide the kreplach among 4 plates, freshly grate the
bottarga on top and serve hot.

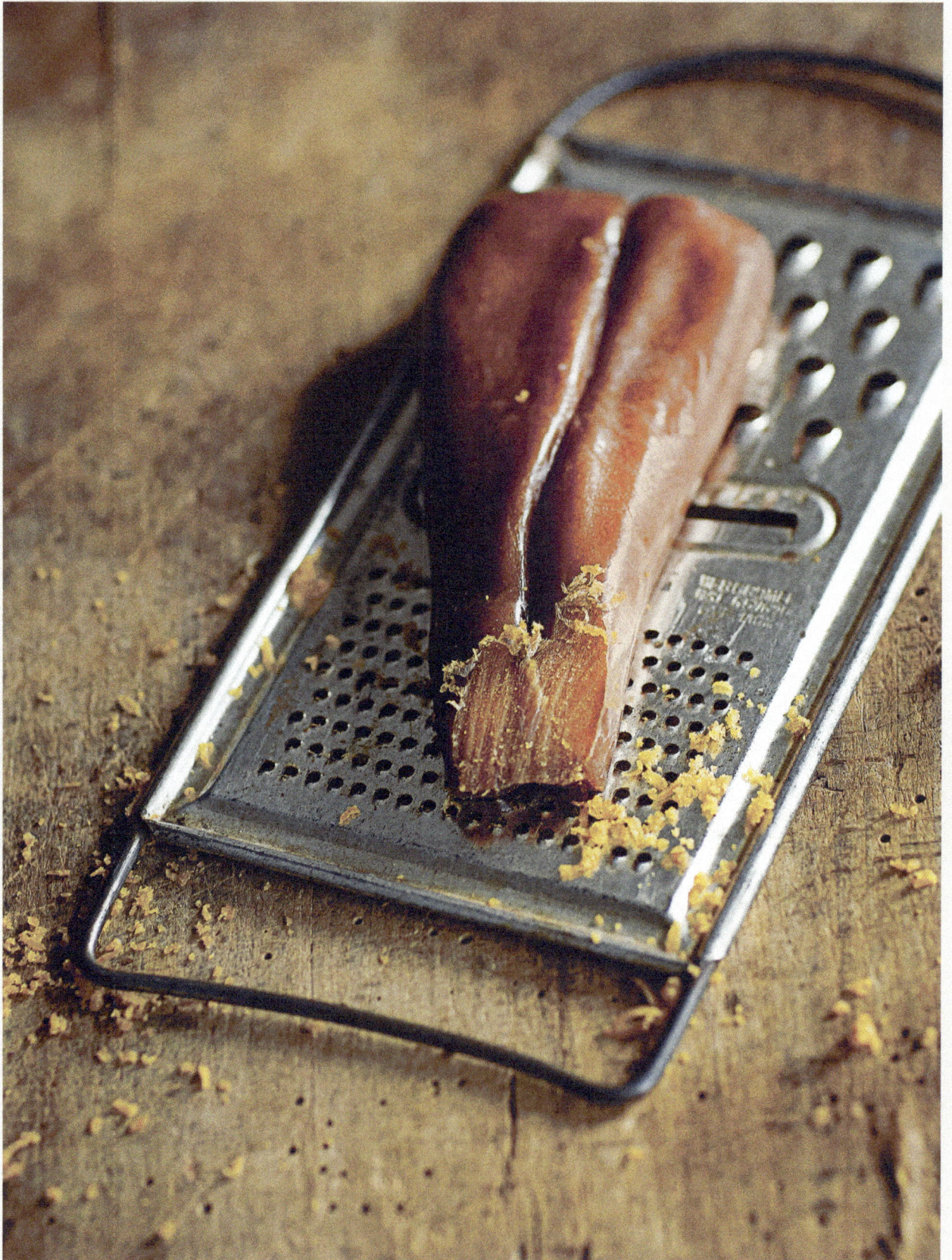

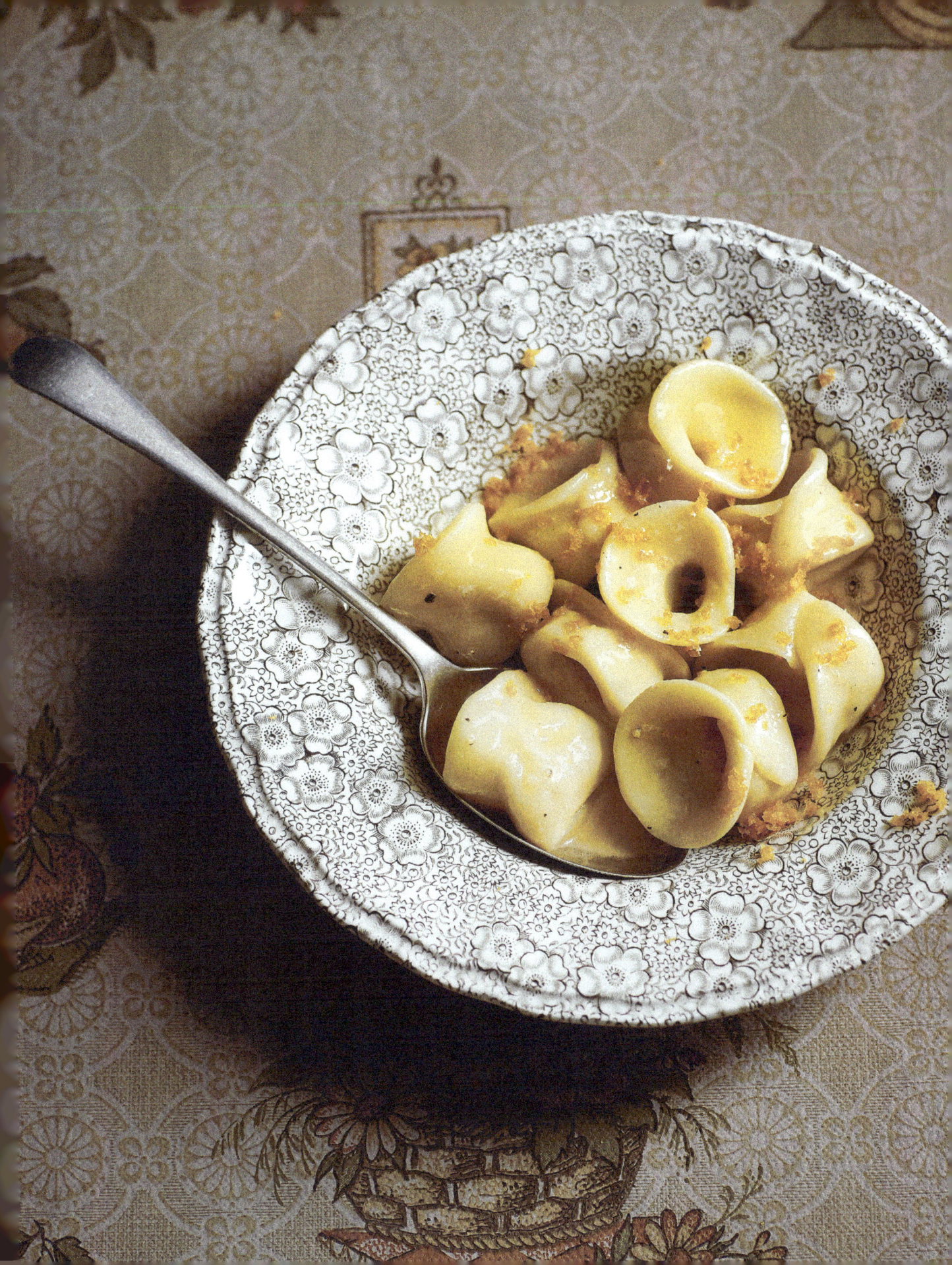

ADEENA SUSSMAN,
Tel Aviv

FAMILY RECIPES,
FAMILY HISTORY

When it comes to cooking, is there anything that Adeena Sussman can't do? Dividing her time between the United States and Israel, the American-born Adeena creates recipes; writes about food for numerous publications; has co-authored numerous cookbooks; and recently published her own cookbook, Sababa: Fresh, Sunny Flavors From My Israeli Kitchen, which the New York Times singled out as "one of the cookbooks you need for 2020."

Adeena grew up in an Orthodox Jewish household in Palo Alto, California. She developed a love for cooking from a young age. In her neighborhood, there were only a few Jewish families, which is why she made a lot of things herself that other people could just pick up at the supermarket. From challah to dessert, in the Sussman household everything was homemade. Part of the reason that Adeena and her sister helped out in the kitchen was because their mother worked outside

the home. One favorite source of inspiration was the New York Times cookbook, from which she ventured to bake such things as a chocolate layer cake. She had two Jewish grandmothers. One loved to cook: from kugel to mandel bread to gefilte fish. The other cooked only once a year for Hanukkah. She made excellent latkes. After graduation, Adeena moved to Israel, where she learned to love seasonal cooking shaped by what was available at the markets. She then got a job at Gourmet Magazine and learned about publishing. She now works freelance as a food writer, recipe and product developer, and consultant.

Food has always played a big part in Adeena's life and she's always asking: what are we eating next? Her devout upbringing meant that her family has spent a lot of time around the table, for Sabbat or holidays. This tradition is important to Adeena and she has integrated it into her own life.

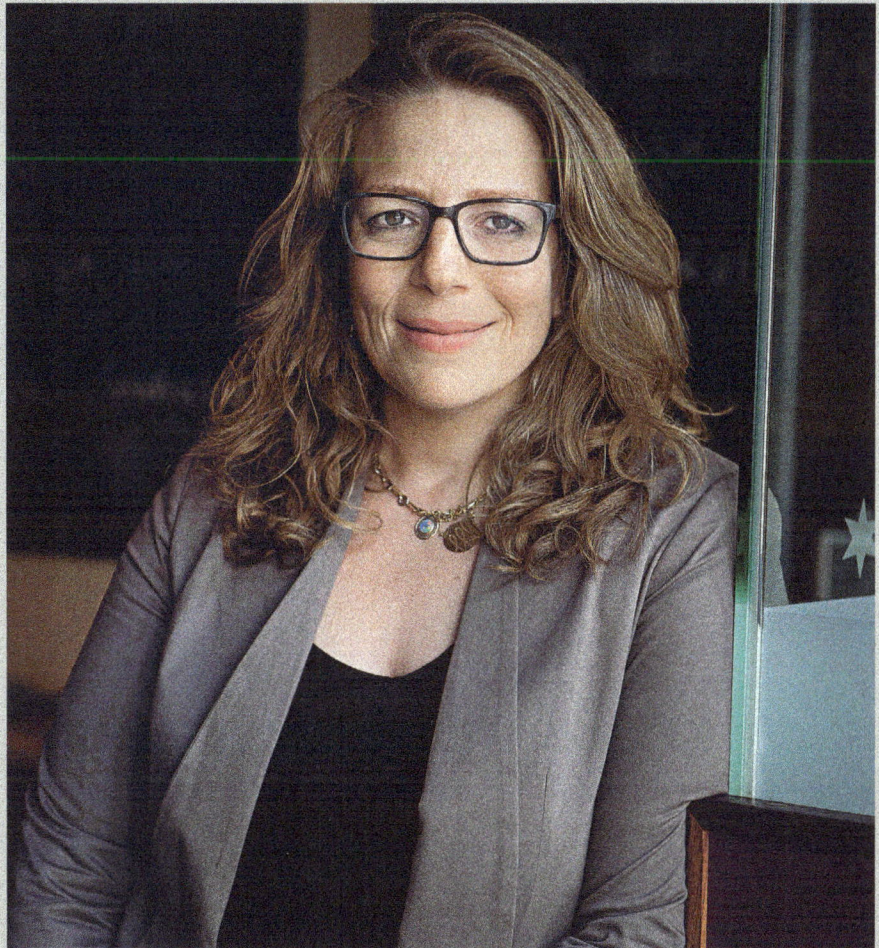

A California native, Adeena divides her time between the US and Tel Aviv. One of her favorite activities is tracking down fresh vegetables at Shuk Ha'Carmel (Carmel Market) in Tel Aviv.

Childhood memories have had a big impact on her relationship to food. Her family likes to recount how when she was just two years old, she was stricken with a stomach flu and wasn't supposed to eat anything. But she nonetheless somehow managed to convince her bubbe, or grandma, to feed her dinner anyway. She also fondly recalls her first Israeli falafel, which she had when she was nine years old. She can still taste it: the crunchy texture of the fried ball, the lusciousness of the tahini, and the crispness of the lettuce. She also recounts with tenderness her deceased mother, Stephanie Ellen Sussman, and how she used to improvise in the kitchen: "Back then, we didn't know what parchment paper was, so my mom would just take a pair of scissors, cut big rectangles out of brown paper bags and use those as a base for her delicious chocolate chip cookies and walnut meringues."

Today, we expect everything to happen instantaneously. Even our memories are recorded, uploaded, and then disappear within 24 hours. In this context, family recipes are even more essential. They provide a connection with something lasting. "I am so grateful that people are taking the time to document our history through food. A million stories lead to an archive of traditions and flavors that future generations can draw from. In some ways, our numbers are dwindling, but through recipes and other edible cultural endeavors, traditions will live on, long after we're gone."

POTATO KUGEL

SERVES 4
PREPARATION: 75 MIN.

POTATO KUGEL
2 tablespoons butter,
    softened
3 ½ lb (1.5 kg) potatoes
1 large onion
4 eggs
1 pinch of freshly ground
    nutmeg
Salt
Freshly ground black
    pepper

This dish is as surprisingly simple as it is delicious. It can be served as an appetizer or side dish. You can try different versions by adding ingredients like cheese (such as Gouda or Emmental) or white cabbage.

POTATO KUGEL
1. Preheat the oven to 350°F. Grease a 9 x 13-inch baking pan with softened butter.
2. Peel and roughly grate the potatoes and onion. Mix the vegetables with the eggs. Add the nutmeg and season generously with salt and freshly ground pepper.
3. Put the potato mixture into the buttered baking pan, smooth it out a bit and bake for about 1 hour until golden brown.
4. Cut into pieces and serve hot.

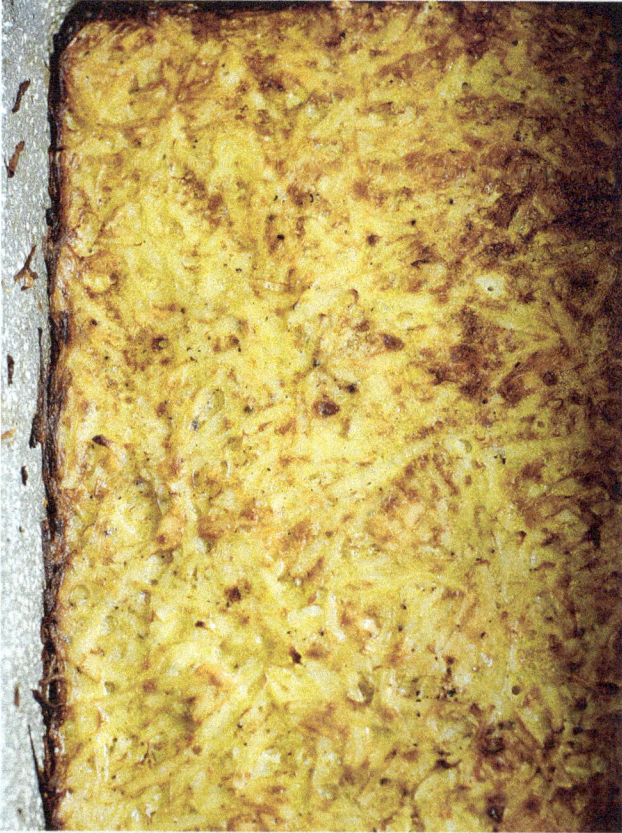

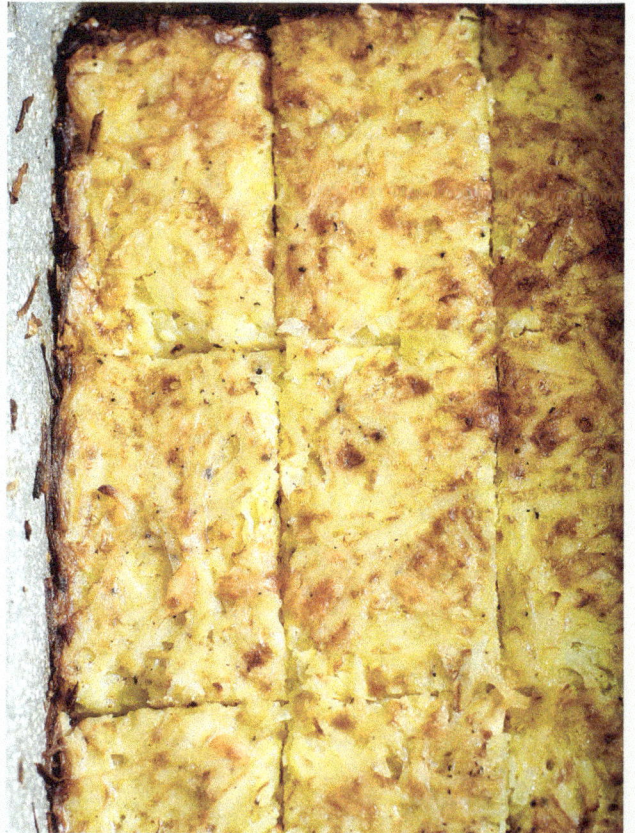

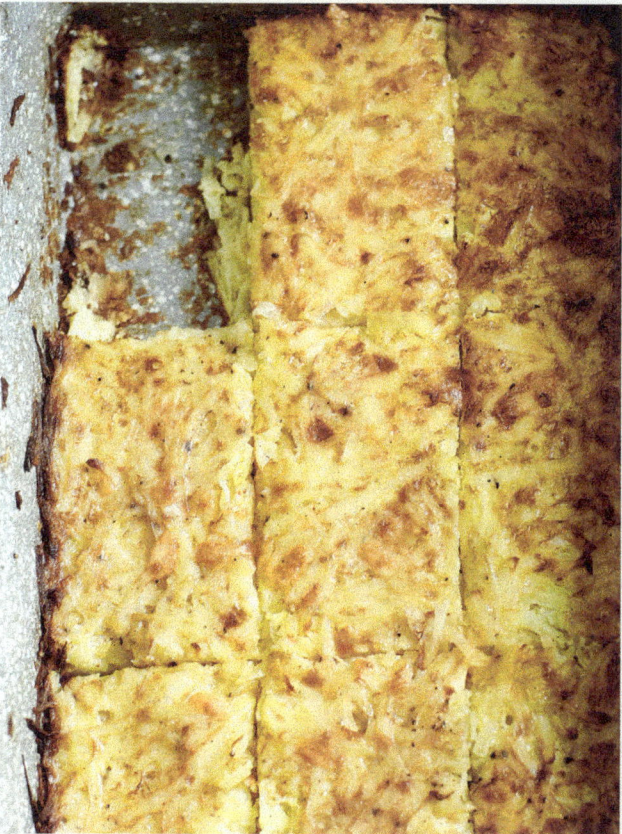

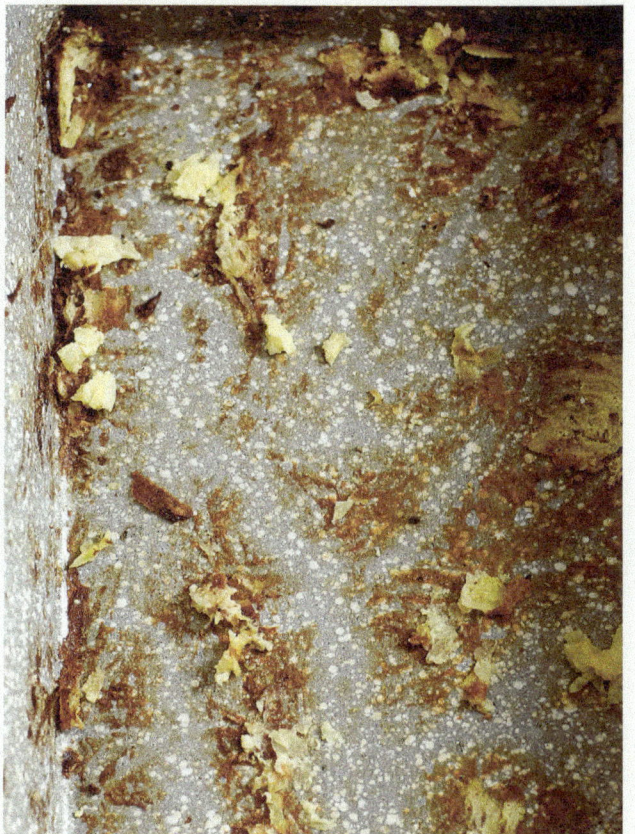

TARAMA
—FISH ROE CREAM

SERVES 4
PREPARATION: 15 MIN.

FISH ROE CREAM
2 slices of white bread,
    toasted and crust re-
    moved
5 ½ oz (150 g) smoked cod
    roe
Plenty of sunflower oil
Salt
Juice from 1 lemon

STOCK
Fresh dill

FISH ROE CREAM
Soak the toasted bread in cold water, squeeze vigorously and place in a blender or food processor together with the roe. Purée the mixture on low speed, adding sunflower oil at first drop by drop, then in a thin stream, until it has a mayonnaise-like consistency. Season the tarama with salt and lemon juice.

Tip: If you cannot get smoked roe, you can use 3 ½ ounces (100 g) smoked salmon and 1 ¾ ounces (50 g) trout caviar. However, the smoky flavor of the roe is unique and therefore worth tracking down.

TO SERVE
Pour the tarama into a small bowl and garnish with some dill. Season with salt and lemon juice and garnish with some dill.

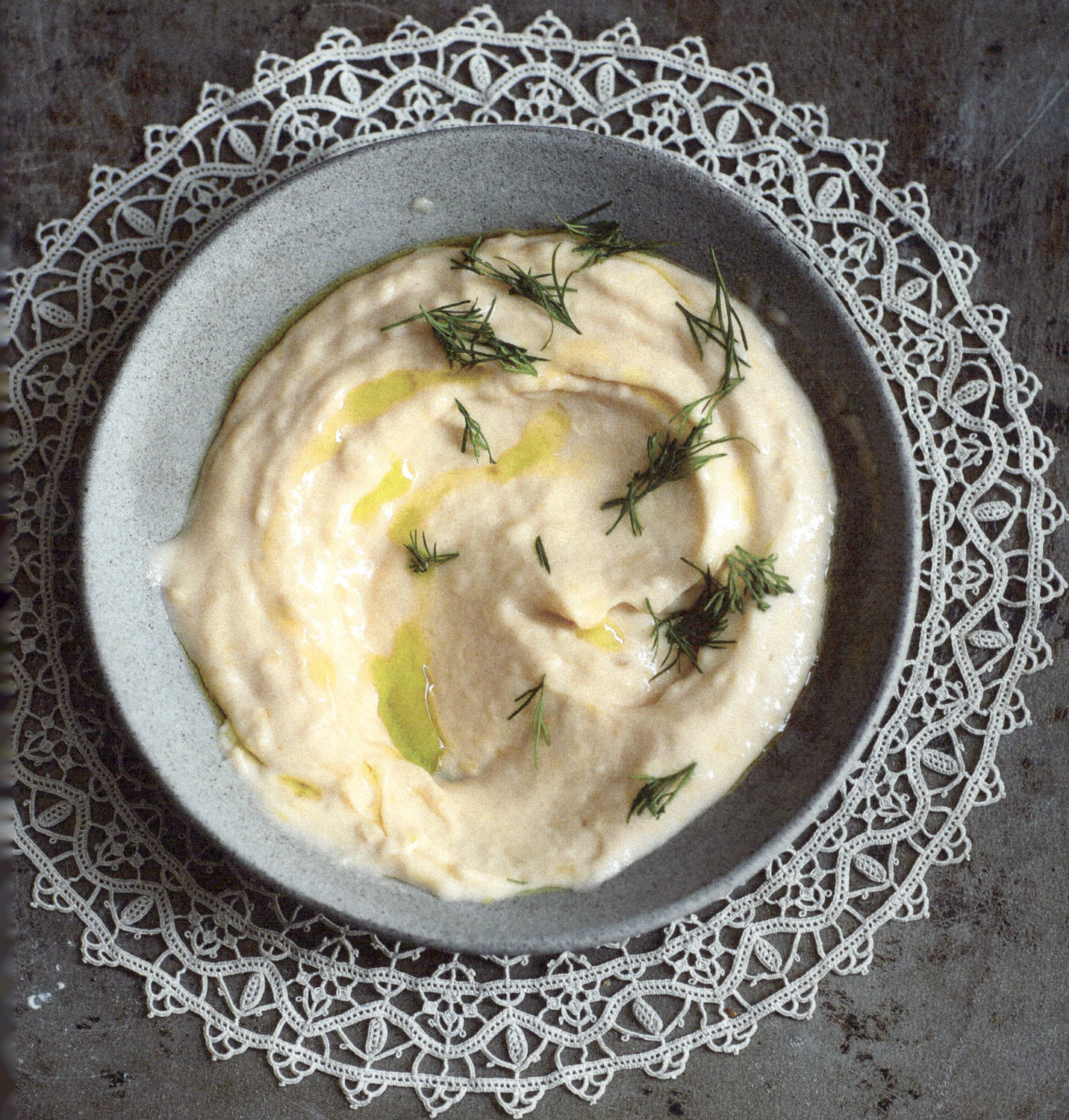

COLD CHERRY SOUP

SERVES 4
PREPARATION: 30 MIN.

CHERRY SOUP
2 lb (1 kg) fresh cherries
1 cup (200 mL) rosé wine
   or dry white wine
1 organic lemon
½–1 cup (100–200 g) sugar
¼ tonka bean, grated
1 tablespoon cornstarch

TO SERVE
½ cup (100 g) crème
   fraîche

CHERRY SOUP

1. Wash and pit the cherries and put them in a pot. Add the wine. Wash the lemon with hot water, using a vegetable peeler, peel off 2 wide strips and add to the pot. Add ½ cup (100 g) of sugar and some grated tonka bean and bring everything to a boil in a pot with a lid on top. If needed, depending on the sweetness of the cherries, add a little more sugar.

2. Let the soup simmer for 5–10 minutes until the cherries are soft. Mix the cornstarch with 2 tablespoons of cold water until smooth and gradually add to the boiling soup, stirring until the liquid thickens slightly. Remove from heat, remove the lemon peel, and let the soup cool.

TO SERVE

Divide the cold cherry soup into 4 bowls and serve with a dollop of cold crème fraîche.

Tip: In summer, the soup makes for a refreshing dessert. However, it can also be prepared warm in cold months, in which case frozen cherries can stand in for fresh ones.

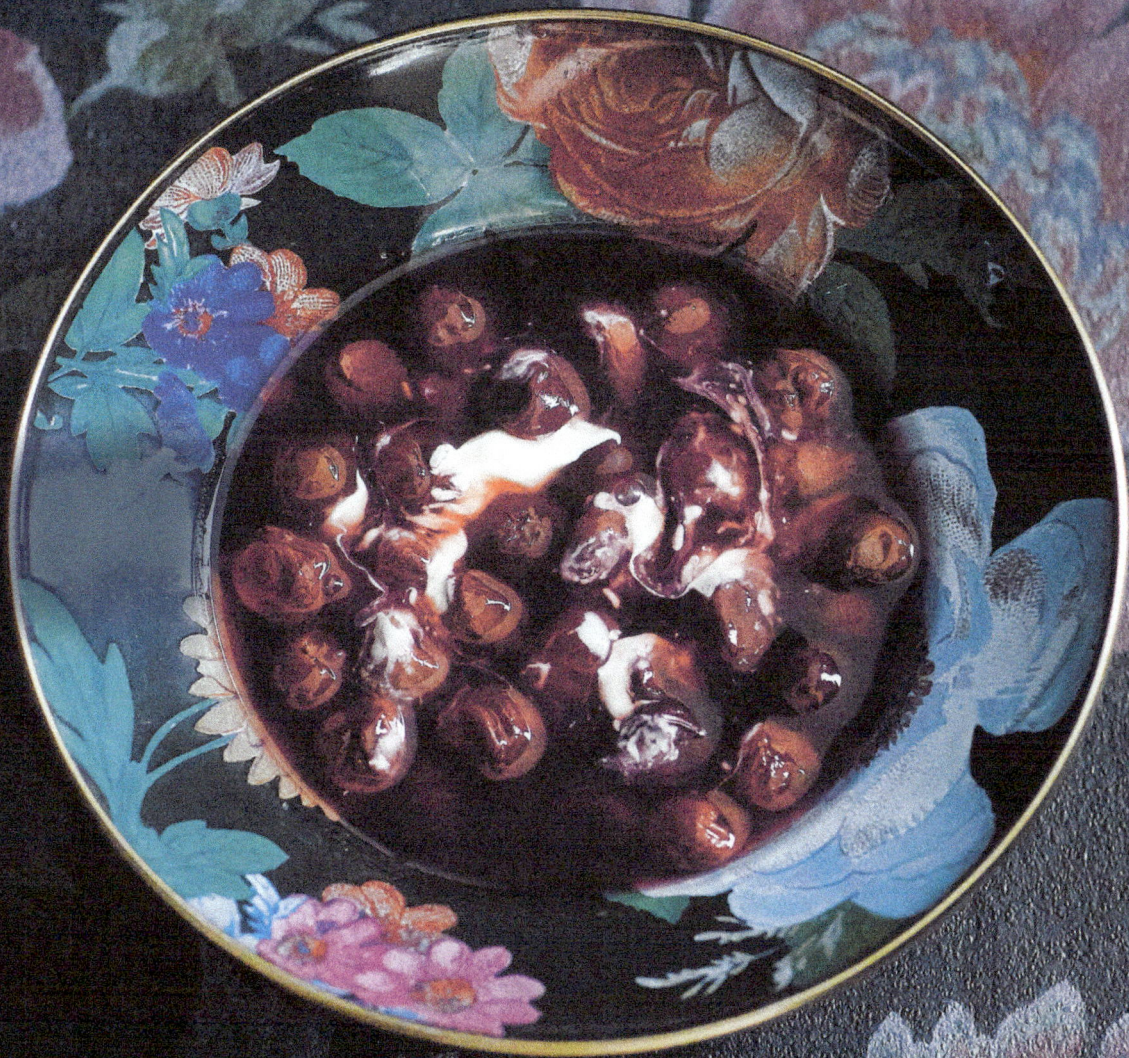

URI SCHEFT, Tel Aviv

ISRAEL'S MOST FAMOUS BAKER

Uri Scheft is probably Israel's most famous baker. His Lehamim Bread Bakery can now be found in Tel Aviv and New York. Born in Israel to Danish parents, in his bakery he makes a wide assortment of baked goods. Uri grew up in Israel and Denmark and spent his summers in Europe; European baking practices have clearly influenced his own.

Uri's been interested in food for as long as he can remember. His mother was a kindergarten teacher who baked challah every Friday. He's always taken inspiration from her skilled baking and the other dishes she used to prepare for Sabbat. Growing up, the whole family would often get together—and not just for the holidays. Whenever they did, there was always an incredible amount of bread.

In 1973, when Uri was eleven, his parents decided to move back to Denmark for a few years. His exposure to Danish bakeries made a lasting impression. That's in part because in Denmark they offered something different than what was available in Israel, which didn't have many bakeries until a couple of decades ago. In Denmark they also offered cooking and baking classes at school, in which Uri gladly enrolled. He still has recipes from those classes he took in school.

Like a lot of Israelis, after completing his military service, he decided to travel before entering university, and continued to do so on and off in college. After graduating from Tel Aviv University, with a degree in biology, Uri woke up one morning and decided to go back to Denmark to study baking. He flew to Copenhagen from India, the latest stop in his travels, with the idea of becoming a pastry chef. He was sure that he'd spend the rest of his life devoted to making pastries. However, because the school didn't have a spot available in their pastry division; they suggested that he turn to their baking school. That's where he realized that baking was his true calling.

After perfecting his baking skills abroad, Uri returned to Israel. In 2002 he opened the bakery Lehamim—"bread" in Hebrew—on Hashmona Street in

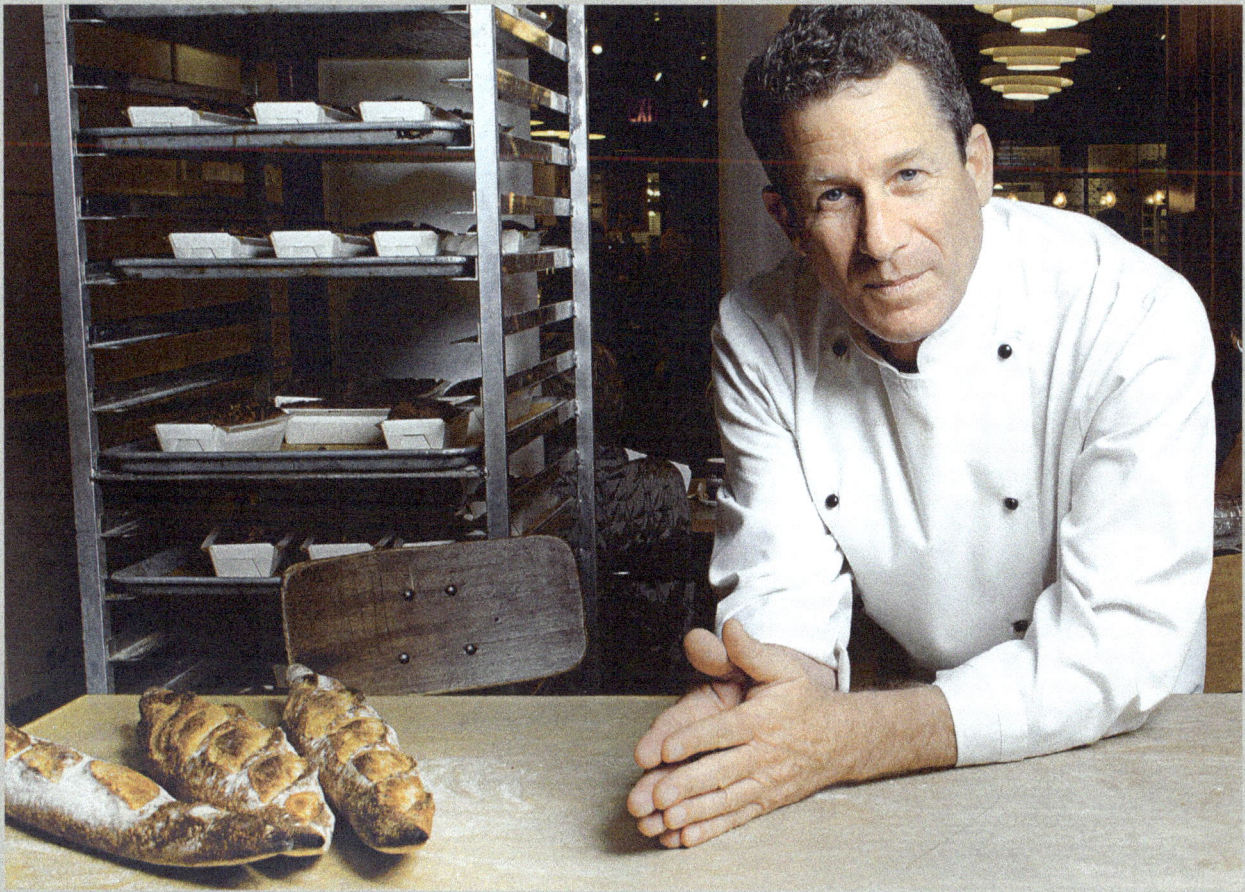

The world-class Israeli baker incorporates his Danish roots into his baking, which can be enjoyed in Tel Aviv and New York.

the heart of Tel Aviv. Lehamim Bakery is open around the clock and closes only on Sabbat. In 2013, Breads Bakery followed in New York City's Union Square, and in the years that followed, he opened two more branches in New York. Uri draws inspiration from many cultures. In addition to his own experience living and traveling in different countries, his grandparents come from Russia, Poland, and Germany. Food from Denmark and Eastern Europe is especially close to his heart and influences his choice of ingredients; he incorporates many of them into the food he makes at home. That extends to the Scandinavian distilled spirit, aquavit, which periodically makes an appearance at his table.

A Danish pastry that Uri particularly likes is the raisin crown. Raisin crowns partner well with tea or coffee. They can also bring a triumphal finish to a good meal. At Uri's Sabbat dinners, you'll find just as much food on the table as there was on his family's when he was growing up. But Uri takes a more modern approach to his recipes. On Fridays, at his house you'll find not only bread, but also lots of salads and Israeli, Danish, and Moroccan-inspired dishes on the table. Uri's wife comes from Morocco and is responsible for the spicy fish dish. What should never be missing? Uri's fresh challah. The challah smell fills the house with a wonderfully warm aroma and will always remind Uri of his mother.

CHALLAH —SABBAT BREAD

SERVES 6 / MAKES 1 LOAF
PREPARATION: 30 MIN.
RISING TIME: 2 - 2 ½ HRS.
BAKING TIME: 45 - 55 MIN.

DOUGH
4 cups (480 g) all-purpose
   flour
2 ¼ teaspoons (7 g) or 1 envelope active dry yeast
¼ cup (60 g) sugar
2 teaspoons salt
2 eggs
1 cup (225 mL) lukewarm water
1 tablespoon neutral vegetable oil

FINAL STEPS
1 egg yolk
2 tablespoons milk
Sesame seeds, poppy seeds,
   and sunflower seeds,
   and coarse sea salt for
   sprinkling, to taste

DOUGH
1. In a large bowl, mix the flour, yeast, sugar, and salt. Form a well in the center, beat the eggs into it and mix with some of the flour. Add the water and, using a wooden spoon, mix the flour with the water from the outside in. Once everything is combined, begin kneading the dough with your hands until it is smooth and pliable, about 10 minutes. Put in a lightly oiled bowl, cover, and let the dough rise in a dark, warm place for 1 ½ - 2 hours until it has doubled in size.
2. Remove the dough from the bowl and divide into 3 equal portions. On a lightly floured work surface, roll each into roughly 1-foot-long strands, weave them into a braid and pinch the ends together. Place on a parchment lined baking sheet and let rise for 30 minutes.

Tip: Experienced bakers can divide the dough into 6 equal portions, roll them into strands and weave a six-link braid.

FINAL STEPS
1. Preheat the oven to 350°F.
2. Whisk the egg yolk with the milk and brush the braid evenly with it. Sprinkle with sesame seeds, poppy seeds, sunflower seeds, and a little sea salt.
3. Bake for 45-55 minutes, until the bread has turned a shiny brown. Before serving, let cool on a rack for at least 60 minutes.

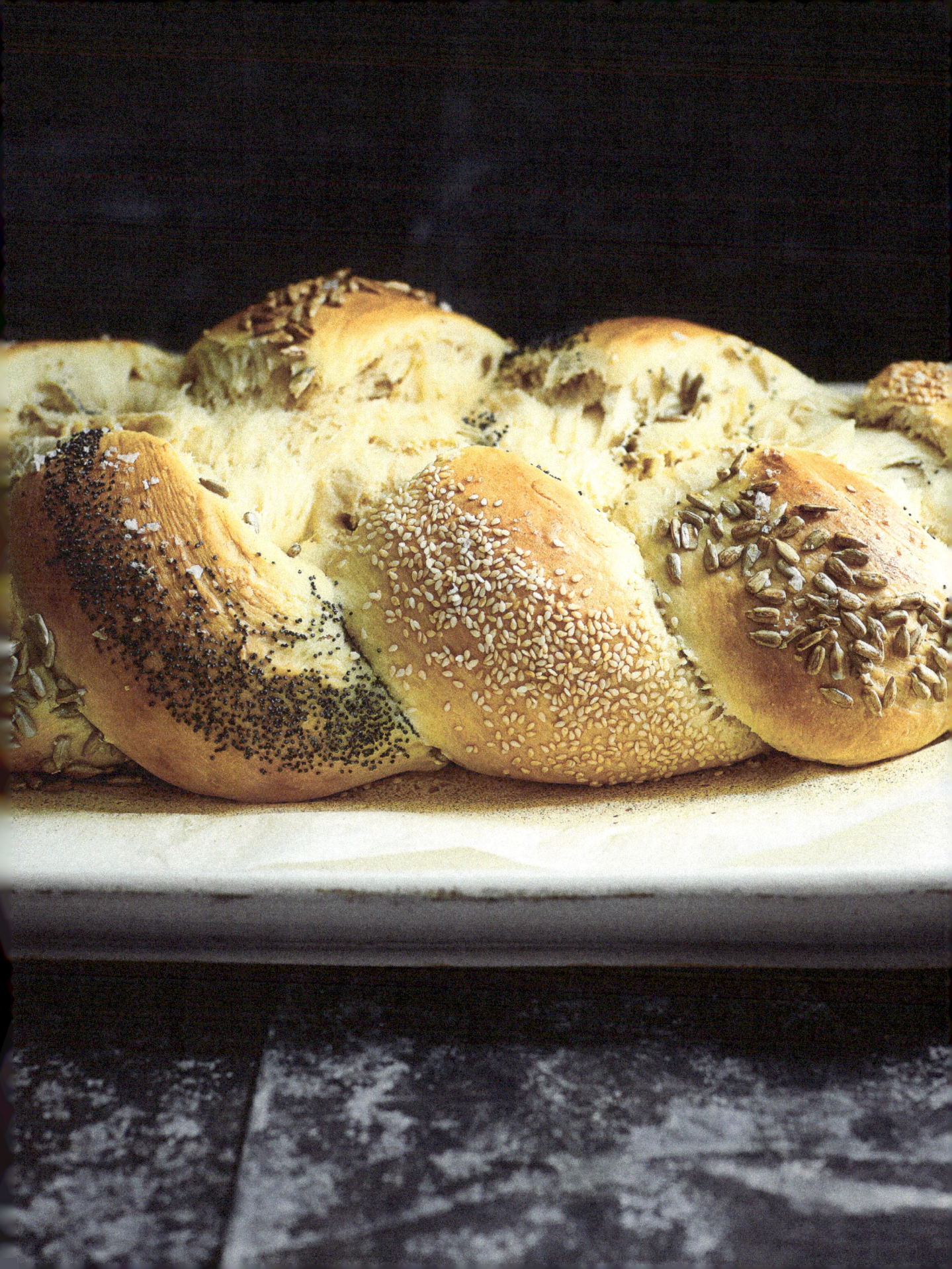

CARAWAY RYE BREAD

MAKES 2 LOAVES
PREPARATION: 30 MIN.
RISING TIME: 2 HRS, 45 MIN.
BAKING TIME: 50 MIN

BREAD
2 ½ cups (500 mL) dark beer
1 ½ teaspoon active dry yeast
4 cups (500 g) rye flour
4 cups (500 g) all-purpose flour
2 2/3 teaspoons (16 g) salt
½ cup (125 mL) lukewarm water
3 teaspoons caraway seeds
Wheat flour or rye flour for work
  surface
Sunflower seeds, and coarse sea
  salt for sprinkling, to taste

BREAD

1. In a small saucepan, heat the beer to a lukewarm temperature and dissolve the dry yeast in it. In a bowl, combine the 2 flours, add the beer, and mix thoroughly. Cover and let it rise for 60 minutes.

2. Dissolve the salt in lukewarm water and add, along with the caraway seeds, to the dough. Using your hands, knead everything until you get a slightly sticky but homogeneous dough. Cover the bowl and let rise for another 60 minutes.

3. Transfer dough to a lightly floured work surface, divide in half and flatten each piece slightly. To create a sort of "envelope" shape, pull the bottom of the dough to the left and to the right, to form two "flaps" or arms. Then fold each "flap" or arm so that they overlap slightly. Repeat the same step, but this time from the top and bottom. Once the four flaps are touching in the middle, seal at the center. Then turn the dough over, so that the flaps are on the bottom and the smooth part is on top. Using your hands, gently drag the dough across the floured surface, and tuck it as you do, creating a slight tension on the outside. Continue to do so until a round, uniform shape is formed.

4. Dust two bowls lined with a kitchen towel (approx. 8 inches in diameter) with flour and place the dough pieces upside down so that the "seam," or lower, open side, is facing up. Cover with a cloth and let rise for another 45 minutes.

5. Preheat a pizza stone or baking sheet on the second rack from the bottom in the oven to 475°F.

6. Bring 3 cups (700 mL) of water to the boil in a kettle or pot. Place a deep baking sheet on the lowest shelf in the oven and carefully pour in the boiling water.

7. Finally, turn the dough out onto the hot pizza stone or baking sheet, score as desired with a sharp knife and bake for 15 minutes. Then remove the bottom tray with the steaming water from the oven, reduce the oven temperature to 400°F and bake for an additional 35 minutes. (Note: The breads are done when they sound hollow on the underside when tapped).

8. Before serving, let cool completely on a rack.

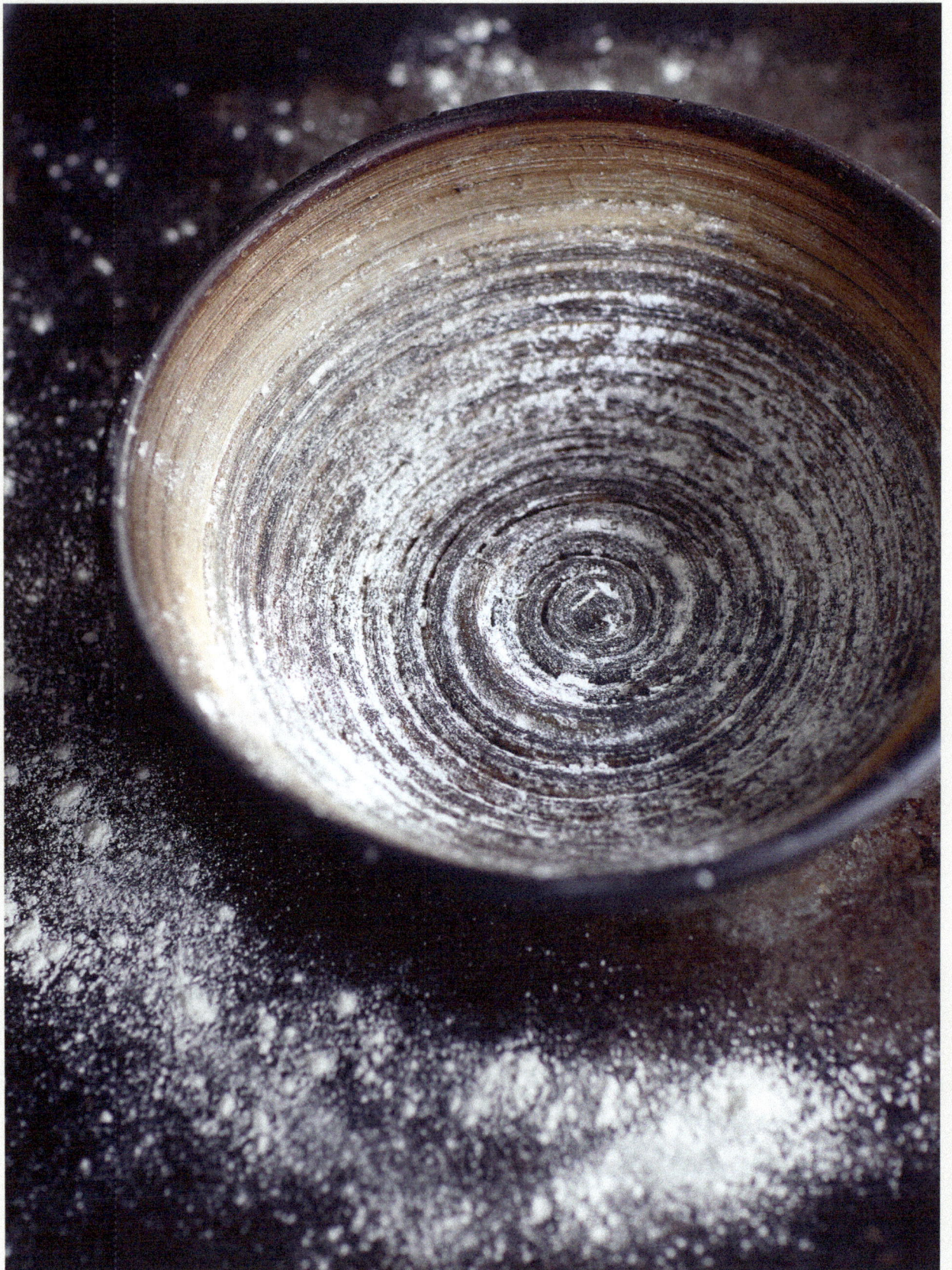

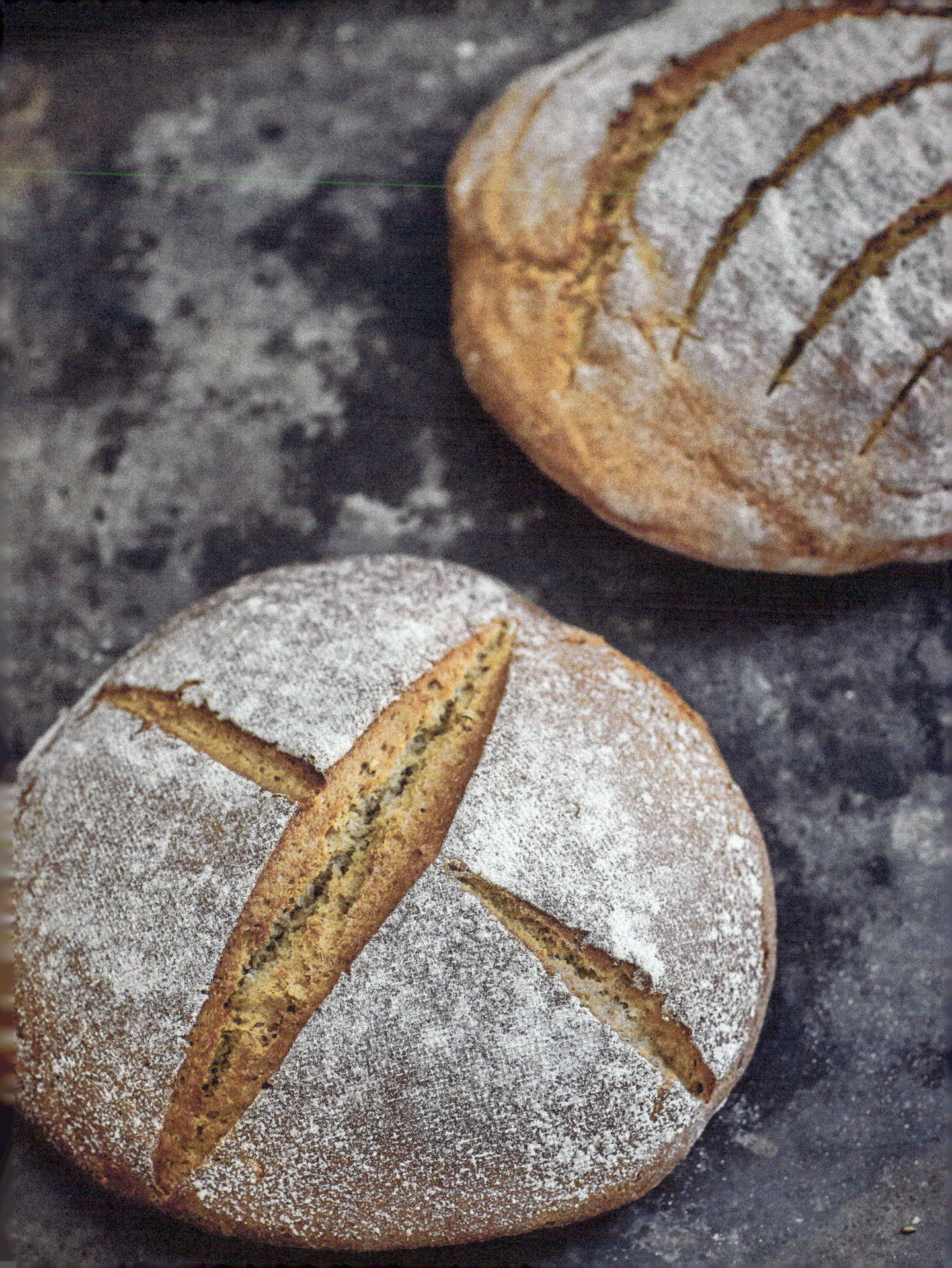

RYE SANDWICH BREAD

MAKES 2 LOAVES
PREPARATION: 30 MIN.
RISING TIME: 13.5 HRS.
BAKING TIME: 60 MIN.

PRE-DOUGH
1 tablespoon (8.5 g) active dry yeast
1 cup (250 mL) lukewarm water
4 tablespoons all-purpose flour
4 tablespoons rye flour

MAIN DOUGH
1 tablespoon (8.5 g) active dry yeast
2 tablespoons honey
1 ½ cups (375 mL) lukewarm water
3 cups (400 g) rye flour
2 ¼ cups (300 g) whole wheat flour
2 ¼ cups (300 g) all-purpose flour
3 1/3 teaspoons (18 g) salt
Some flour for work surface
Some neutral vegetable oil for the pan

PRE-DOUGH

In a bowl, add dry yeast, lukewarm water, the all-purpose and rye flours and mix with a spoon. Cover with a cloth and let rise for 12 hours at room temperature.

MAIN DOUGH

1. Dissolve the dry yeast and honey in the lukewarm water. In a large bowl, mix the flours and salt. Add the pre-dough and the yeast-honey-water and knead everything for 5 minutes until a homogeneous dough is formed. Cover and let rise for 60 minutes until doubled in size.

2. Transfer the dough to a lightly floured work surface, divide in half and flatten each piece slightly. Fold each piece of dough first from the left and right, then from the top and bottom toward the center, turning the dough once so that the smooth, closed side is on top. Using your hands, gently work the dough in circular motions so that a slight tension is created on the upper side. Do not continue to knead or fold the dough, merely give it shape.

3. Turn the rounded dough pieces over and gently roll them up into oblong loaves, with the seam facing inward. Place the loaves, seam side down, in lightly oiled medium loaf pans, cover and let rise in a warm, dark place for 30 minutes until about doubled in size.

4. Preheat the oven to 350°F.

5. Spritz the loaves with a generous amount of water and bake for 50 minutes. Remove the loaves from the loaf pans while still hot and bake for an additional 10 minutes on a baking sheet. Before serving, cool on a rack for at least 60 minutes.

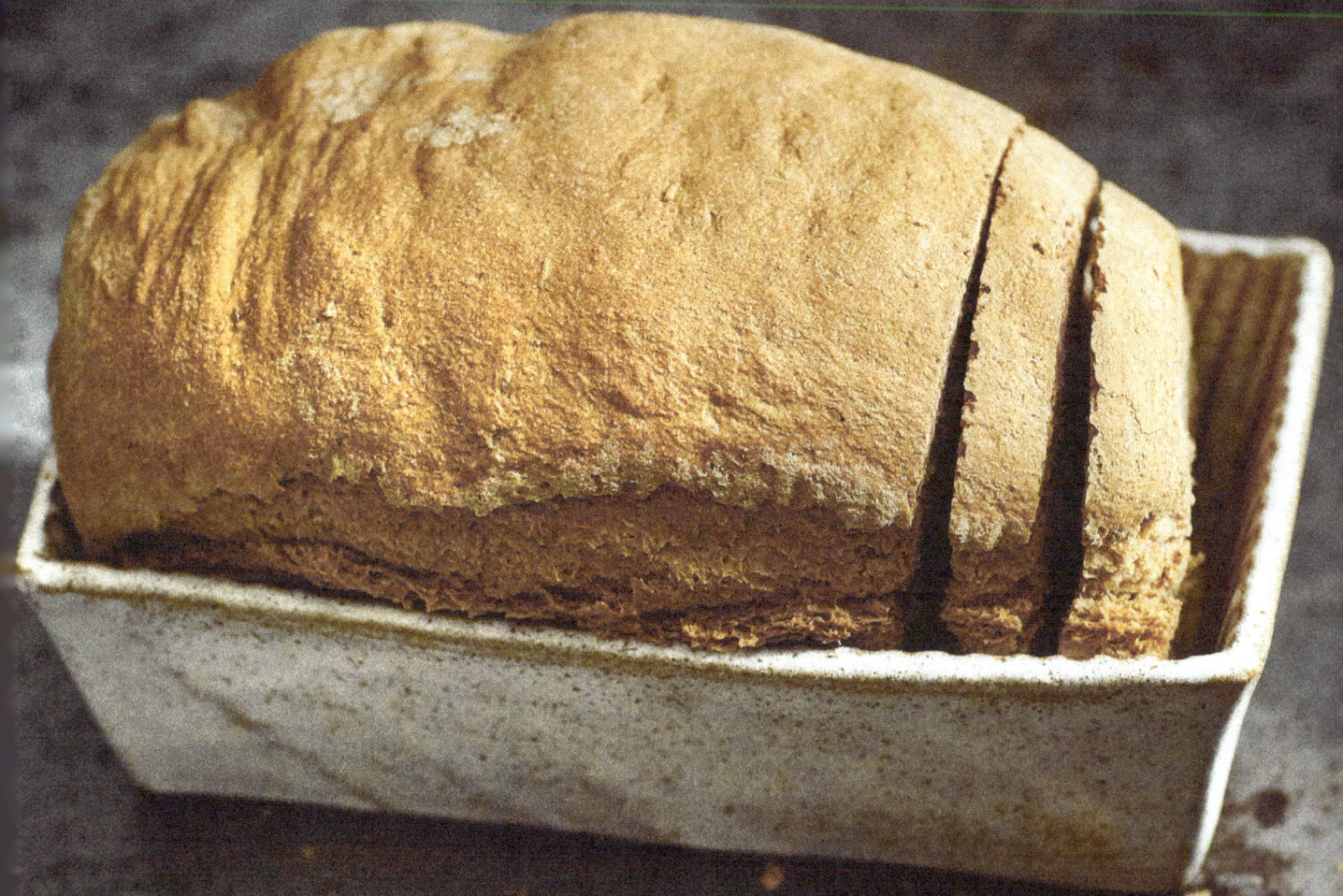

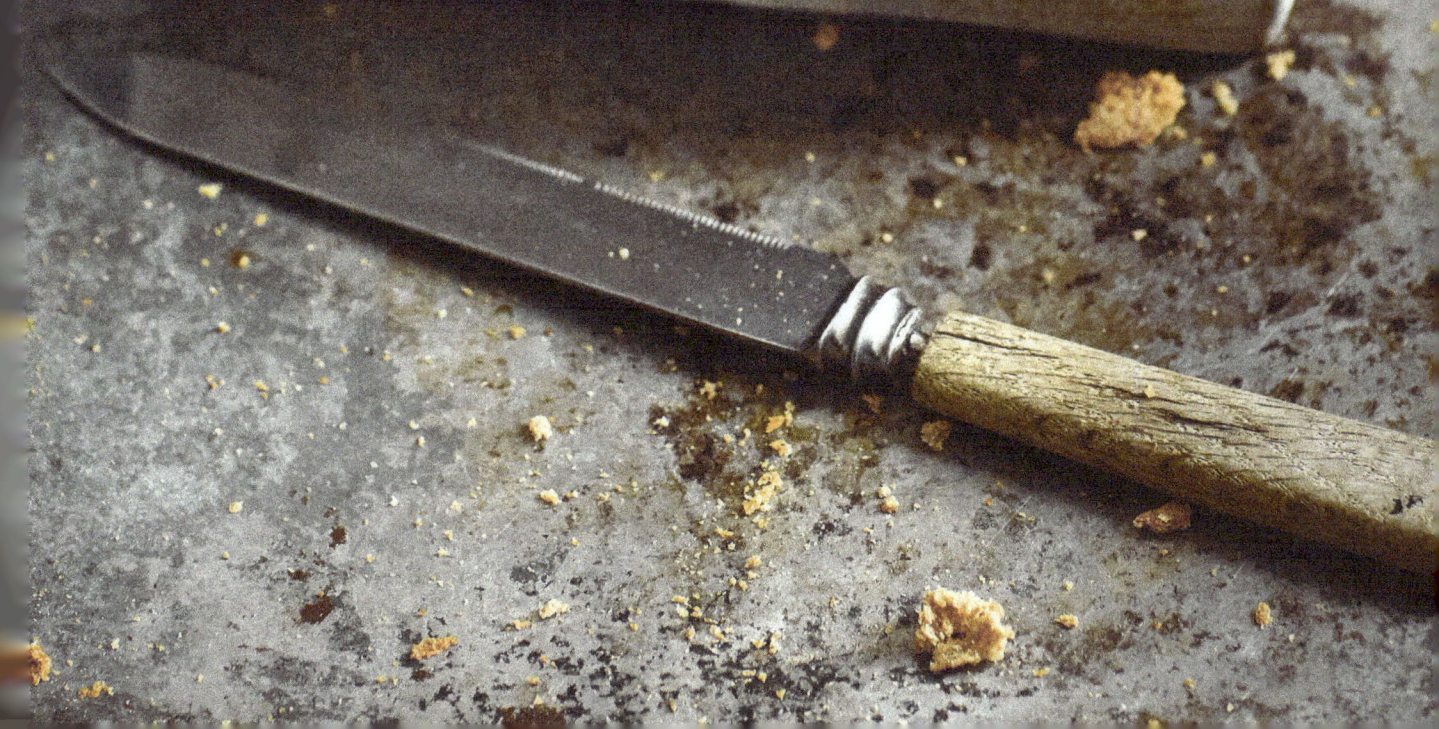

RAISIN CROWNS

SERVES 6 / 1 LARGE CROWN WITH 8 ROLLS
PREPARATION: 20 MIN.
RISING TIME: 90 MIN.
BAKING TIME: 30 MIN.

DOUGH

1 tablespoon (9 g) active dry yeast
1 ¼ cups (300 g) lukewarm water
4 3/4 cups (600 g) pastry flour
1 pinch of salt
¼ cup (50 g) sugar
3 ½ tablespoons (50 g) butter, softened
¾ cup (150 g) raisins

FINAL STEPS

Flour for work surface
1 tablespoon butter, softened
1 egg
2 tablespoons water

DOUGH

1. In a large bowl, dissolve the yeast in the lukewarm water. Gradually add flour, salt, sugar, and butter. Knead into an elastic dough, about 10 minutes. Finally, knead in the raisins.

2. Turn the dough out onto a lightly floured work surface and form into a ball. Put back into the bowl, cover and let rise in a warm, dark place for 30 minutes.

FINAL STEPS

1. Remove from bowl and divide into 8 equal portions. Dust the work surface with a little flour. Using the hollow of your hand, roll each portion of dough into a ball. Then working in circular motions and with gentle pressure, continue to work the dough until the top is closed and slightly taut. Dust the work surface again with flour, place the balls of dough on it, cover with a cloth and let rise for another 30 minutes.

2. Grease a springform pan (10-inch diameter) with softened butter. Place the balls of dough in the pan, forming a crown, cover and let rise for another 30 minutes.

3. Meanwhile, preheat the oven to 350°F.

4. Whisk the egg and the water and brush the raisin crown with it. Bake for 25-30 minutes until golden brown. Remove from oven.

5. Before serving, let cool on a rack for at least 30 minutes.

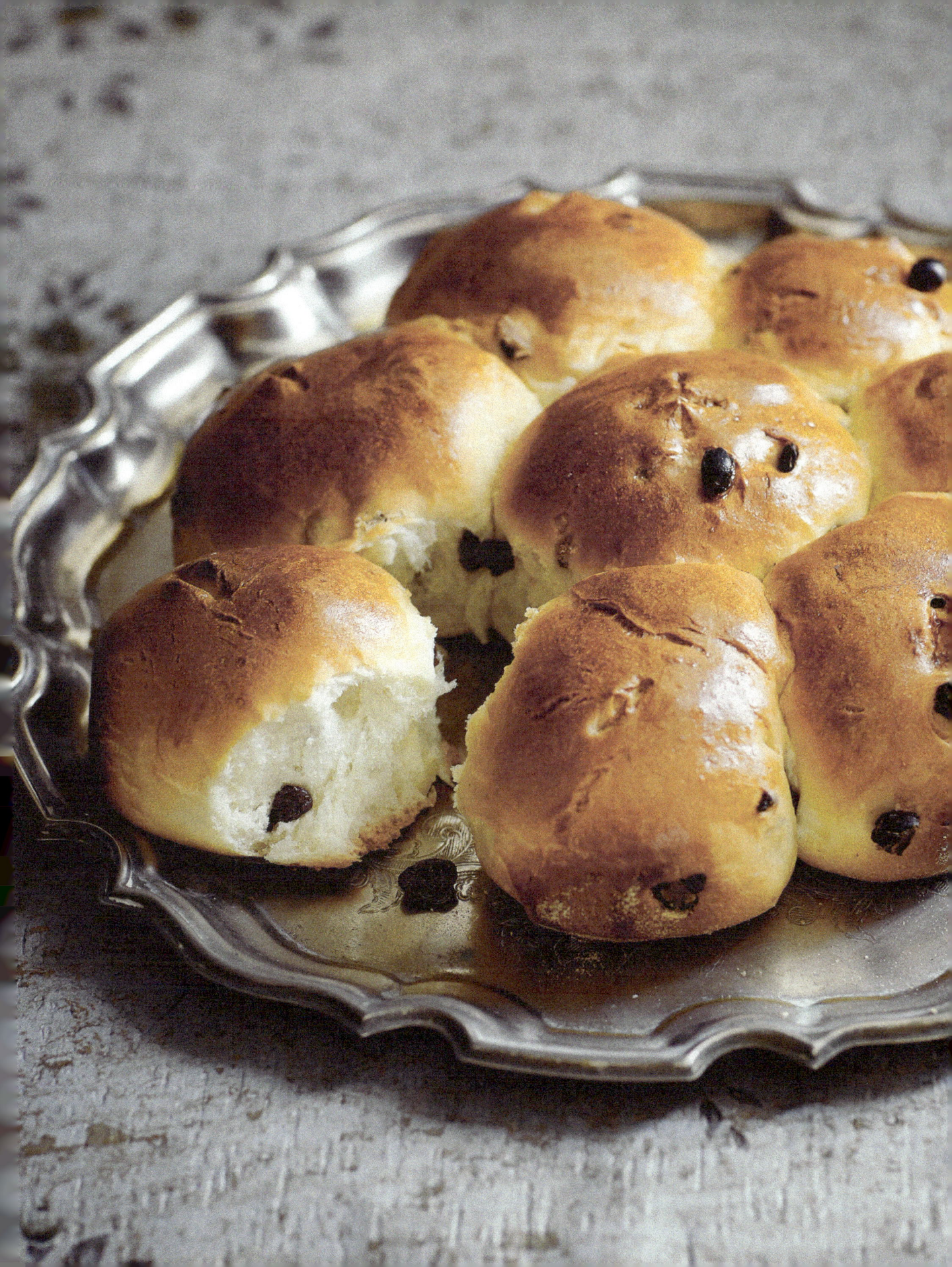

AVI AVITAL, Tel Aviv

FOOD AS IDENTITY AND HOME

Avi Avital is a well-traveled Israeli mandolinist and composer with Moroccan roots. The diaspora has greatly impacted his identity. Both of his parents are from Morocco and his last name, Avital, is a common Israeli-Moroccan one. Like a lot of immigrants to Israel, when his parents arrived their goal was to be part of a new, homogeneous civil society. To fit in, a lot of immigrants change their last names to sound more Israeli. But his family chose not to, which had a fundamental influence on Avi's childhood, as his origins were never hidden from view. Avi views Israel with nuance. Some things have worked really well there, some haven't. But one thing is certain: although it may be complicated to reconcile differences, the diversity of humanity is a beautiful thing. Avi experienced such diversity firsthand, at his school, where a lot of kids had parents who weren't born in Israel.

Cultural identity, Avi observes, is strongly tied to food. In his home, for instance, they maintained their ties to Morocco through food, not through language—Avi regrets that his parents didn't pass on Arabic to him. Nor will he ever forget his first, most powerful experiences with the Moroccan-influenced food served at his home and at his grandmother's. His maternal grandmother had eleven children and a lot of grandchildren too. On Fridays after school and before Sabbat, all the grandchildren would come over. In anticipation of Sabbat, all the food was prepared between Thursday evening and Friday morning; on Friday afternoons the cooking would stop. Avi can still clearly remember the chaos of the kitchen filled with uncles and aunts dishing up his grandmother's homemade couscous. All the burners were occupied, and the kitchen was fragrant with various odors. Before dinner, there was freshly baked bread with meatballs to snack on.

Everyone's knows that olives made for a good snack or appetizer. Avi, however, fondly recalls the way his mother used to serve them. Instead of merely dumping

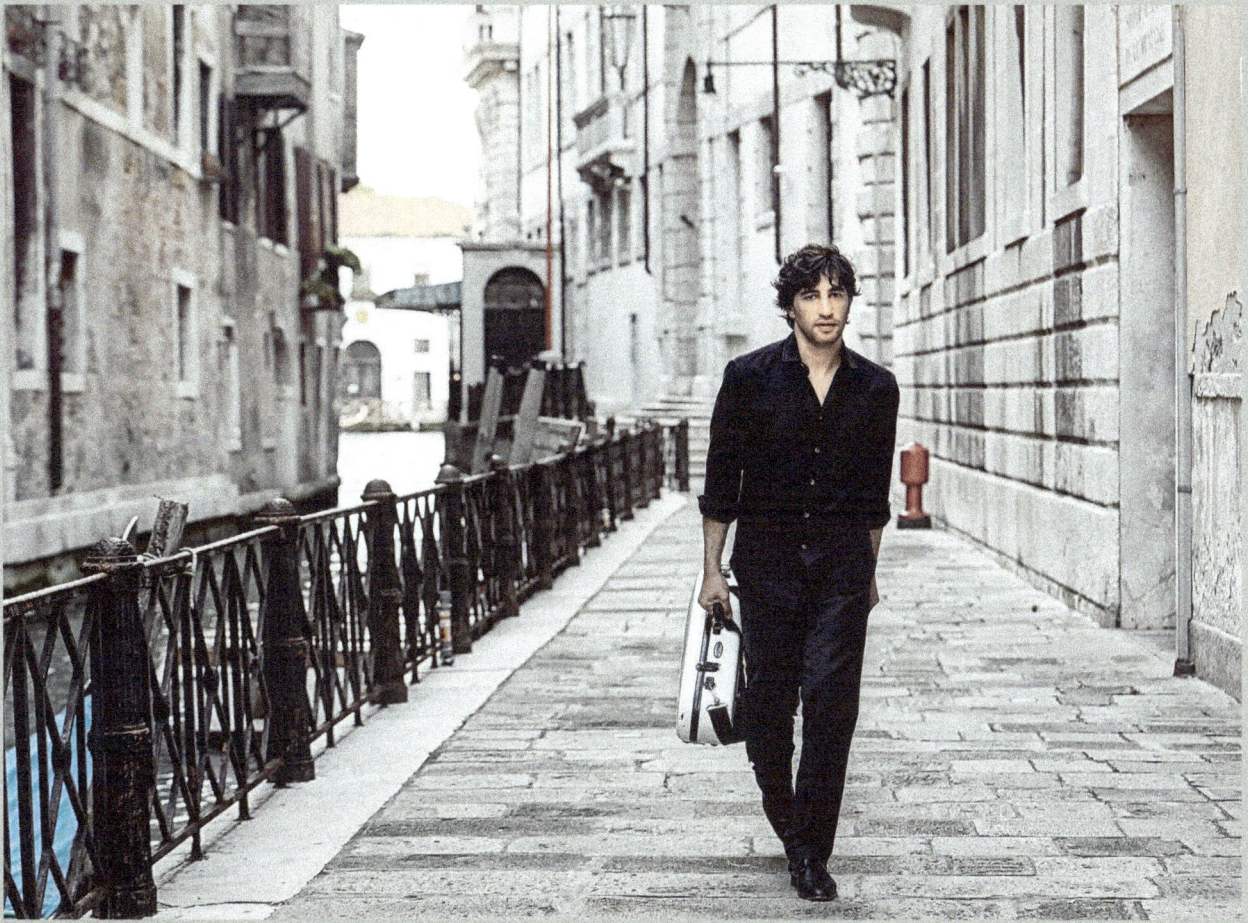

Avi Avital is a professional mandolinist. At home, he's also in charge of the pasta.
(Photo © Harald Hoffmann/Deutsche Grammophon)

them in a bowl, she would cook black olives first with water and lemon and then boil them with tomato paste and various spices. This makes for a delicious sauce that's perfect for dipping bread and a great accompaniment to the first drink.

As a musician, these days Avi spends most of his time on tour and never stays anywhere for more than a week. This makes "home" more of a more spiritual notion than a physical location. He feels at home everywhere. Food, along with music, is a powerful emotional connection to places that he visits and to his past. When he's in Israel, he always makes a number of stops that connect him with the home where he grew up. These include enjoying Sabbat dinner with his parents and when he's in Jerusalem he enjoys falafel, which is one of his favorite things to eat. Because he travels so much, he eats out a lot. So cooking anywhere

can make him feel at home. One dish he loves to prepare is fresh pasta, something he learned to cooked to perfection after living in Milan for many years.

When Avi was a teenager, his friends always wanted to come to his house for dinner. They found Moroccan cuisine more exciting than the Ashkenazi Jewish food that most of their moms made. Perhaps Avi's son will feel the same way one day, but instead of coming over for Moroccan made by his mom, they'll want to come over for Italian pasta made by his dad.

MOM'S ZEITIM —OLIVES IN TOMATO SAUCE

SERVES 4
PREPARATION: 25 MIN.

OLIVES IN TOMATO SAUCE
3 cups (270 g) green pitted
   olives
Juice from ½ lemon
½ cup (100 g) tomato purée
1 teaspoon hot paprika
½ teaspoon ground cumin
4 tablespoons olive oil
Salt
Freshly ground black pepper

TO SERVE
Freshly baked kubaneh (see p.
   18) or challah (see p. 44)

OLIVES IN TOMATO SAUCE
Bring the olives to a boil in a small pot along with the lemon juice. Cover the pot with a lid and simmer gently for 15 minutes. Drain the olives and return to the pot. Add the tomato purée, paprika, cumin, and olive oil. Mix well. Pour in just enough water to cover ingredients and simmer on medium-high heat until sauce has thickened. Season with salt and freshly ground pepper.

TO SERVE
Place the olives and tomato sauce in a bowl. Serve with a piece of freshly baked kubaneh or challah.

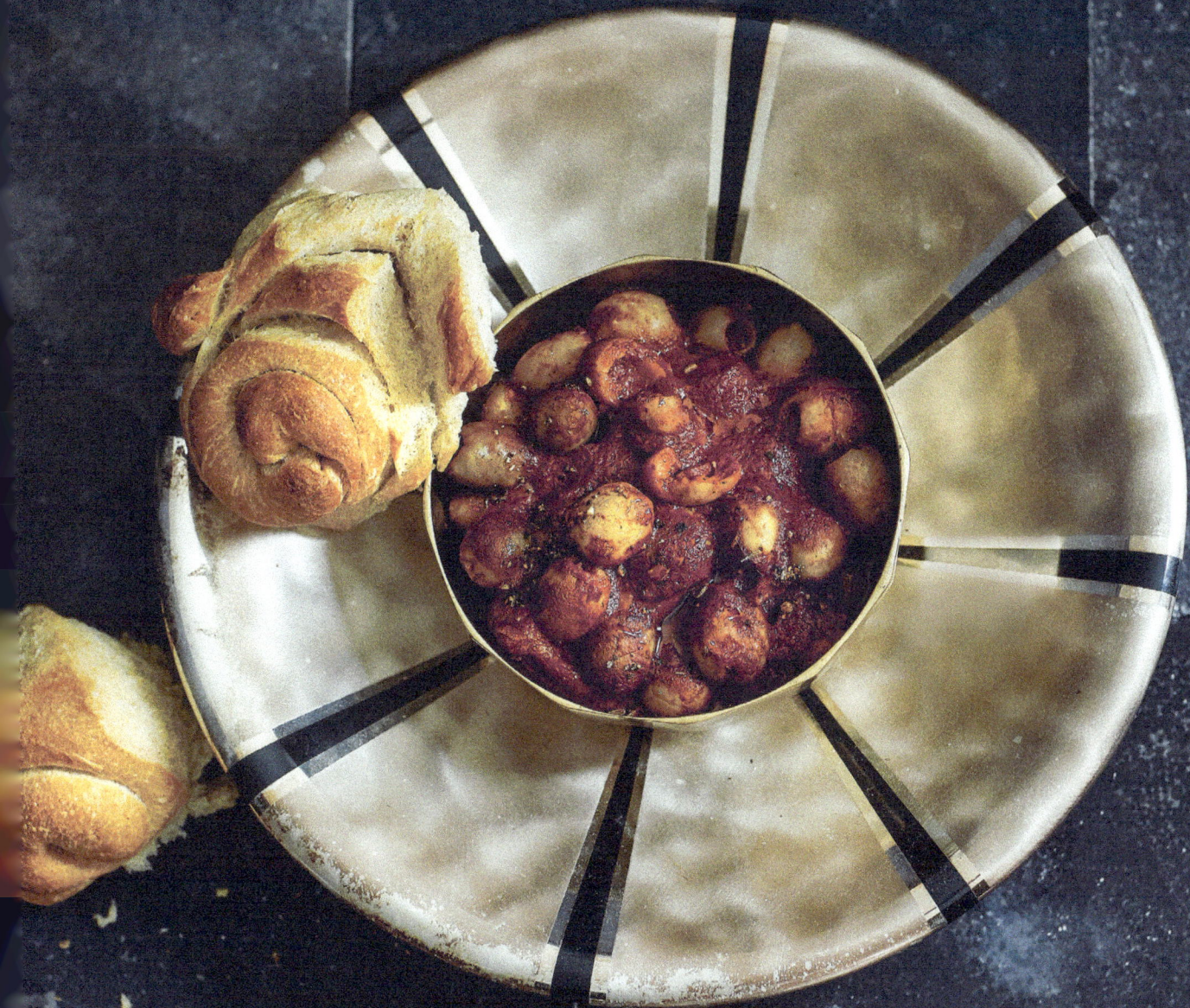

GRANDMA'S MEATBALLS

SERVES 6 / MAKES 18 BALLS
PREPARATION: 45 MIN.

MEATBALLS
2 lb (1 kg) ground beef
1 medium onion
1 large potato
1 small bunch of cilantro
1 egg
Salt
Freshly ground black pepper
2 tablespoons vegetable oil for frying
1 tablespoon sweet paprika
½ teaspoon ground cumin
1 cup (240 mL) water
Some vegetable oil for shaping the balls

TO SERVE
Fresh bread or cooked rice, to taste

MEATBALLS

1. Place the ground beef in a large bowl.

2. Peel and cut the onion in half. Finely dice one half, and set aside. Using a grater, coarsely grate the remaining onion. Peel the potato and grate it coarsely as well.
Mix the grated onion with the grated potato, squeeze vigorously with your hands, and add to the ground beef. Wash the cilantro and chop it along with the stems. Add half of it to the ground beef mixture. Set the remaining cilantro aside.

3. Add the egg to the ground beef mixture. Season everything with salt and freshly ground pepper and mix well.

4. Heat the vegetable oil in a large skillet and sweat the diced onion until translucent. Add the paprika, cumin, salt, and freshly ground pepper and cook for 1 minute. Deglaze the sauce with the water, scraping up the bits clinging to the bottom of the skillet, and bring to a boil, then reduce to a simmer.

5. Meanwhile, with lightly oiled hands, form 18 equal-sized balls from the ground beef mixture. Add the meatballs to the sauce, cover the pan with a lid and cook the meatballs on low for about 20 minutes. Finally, remove the lid and, if necessary, reduce the sauce until it has a thick, creamy consistency. Finally, stir the remaining cilantro into the sauce and season to taste.

TO SERVE
Divide the meatballs among 6 plates and serve with fresh bread or cooked rice, if desired.

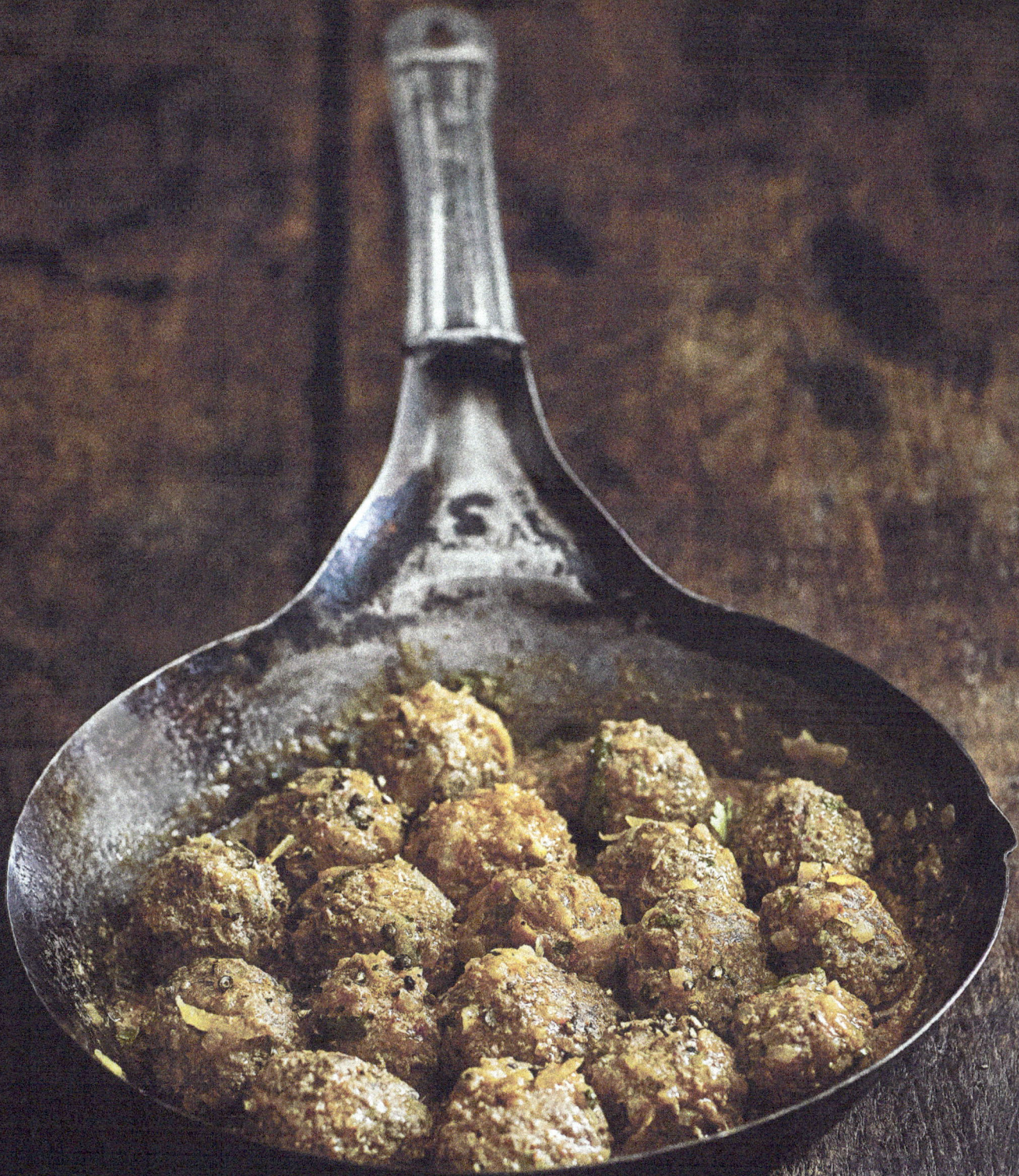

GROUPER—FIG SASHIMI

SERVES 6
PREPARATION: 30 MIN.

GROUPER FIG SASHIMI
6 fresh figs
½ bunch parsley
½ bunch cilantro
2 spring onions
1 fresh red chili pepper
1 lb (500 g) fresh fillet of
    red grouper (grouper,
    alternatively fillet of
    red snapper, skinless,
    sashimi quality)

TO SERVE
6 tablespoons sheep
    yogurt
Coarse sea salt
Freshly crushed black
    peppercorns
Juice from 2 lemons
Some olive oil

GROUPER FIG SASHIMI

1. Preheat a grill or the oven to the highest setting.
2. Wash the figs, pat them dry and grill on all sides for 2-3 minutes. Allow to cool.
3. De-stem parsley and cilantro leaves, wash and pat dry. Then coarsely chop them. Clean the spring onions, cut off the roots and chop into thin rings, then mix them with the herbs. Remove the stalk, seeds, and membrane from the chili pepper and chop into thin rings.
4. Cut the fish into 3/4-inch-wide strips and then into ¼-inch-thin sashimi slices. Cut the grilled figs into ¼-inch-thin slices.

TO SERVE

In the center of each of 6 plates, spoon 1 tablespoon of sheep yogurt and spread lightly with a spoon. Arrange the sashimi slices, figs, and herbs loosely on top, forming a slight curve. Then season everything with coarse sea salt and freshly crushed peppercorns and drizzle with lemon juice and a little olive oil. Finally, garnish with sliced chilis, as desired.

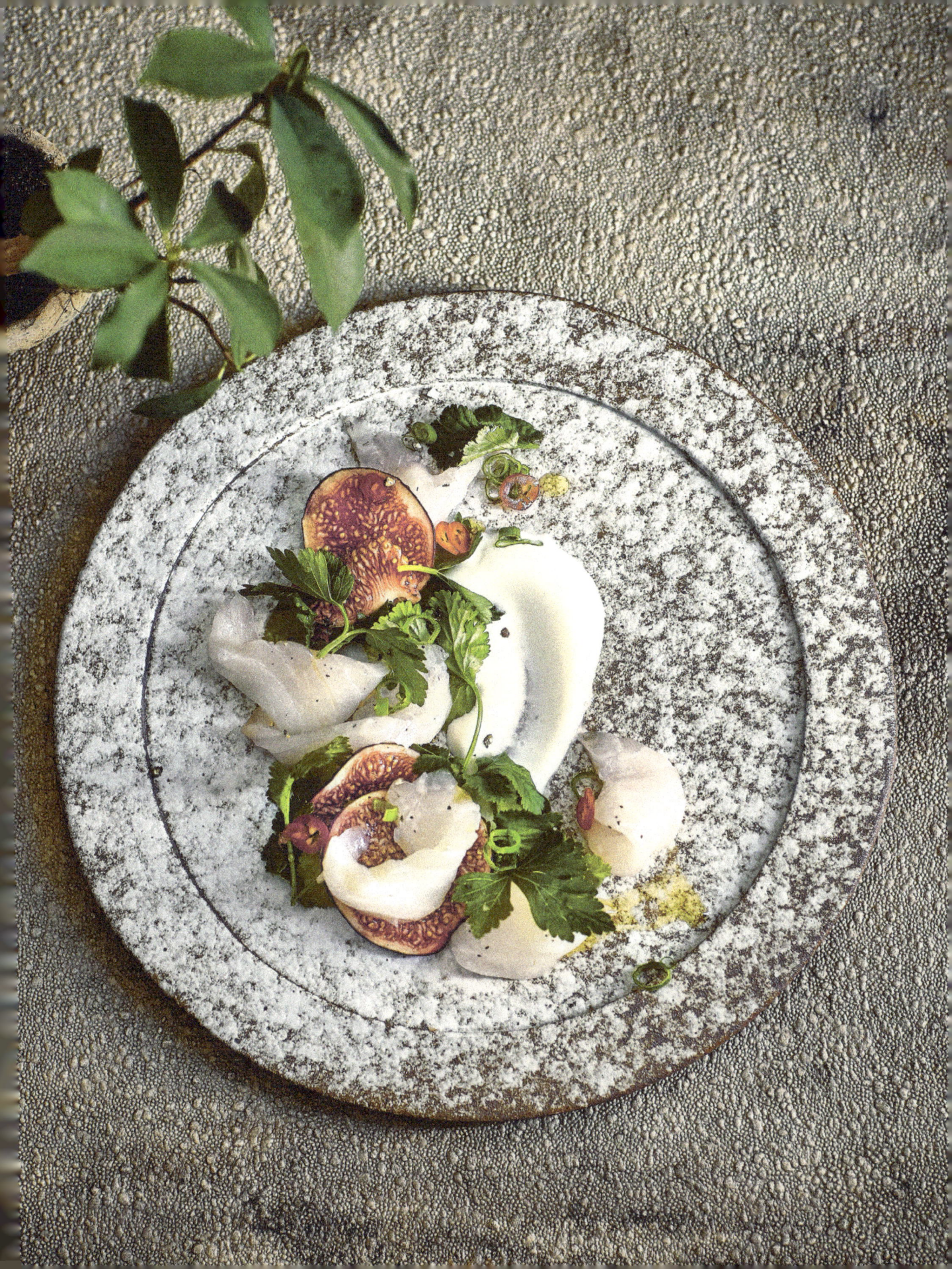

HUNGARIAN CHICKEN STEW WITH AN ISRAELI TOUCH

SERVES 2
PREPARATION: 35 MIN.
MARINATING TIME: 1 HR.
COOKING TIME: 45 MIN.

CHICKEN STEW
2 chicken thighs (8-9 oz /
   250 g each)
Salt
Freshly ground black
   pepper
1 tablespoon sweet paprika
1 red bell pepper
1 yellow bell pepper
1 tomato
1 onion
3 cloves of garlic
1 fresh green chili pepper
1 tablespoon olive oil
1 tablespoon coriander
   seeds, crushed
1 tablespoon date syrup (or
   honey)
¼ cup (50 mL) dry white
   wine
½ cup (100 mL) chicken
   stock

CHICKEN THIGHS
1. Wash the chicken thighs, pat dry and rub with salt, freshly ground pepper, and 1 pinch of paprika and place in a deep bowl. Cover and let marinate in the refrigerator for 1 hour.
2. In the meantime, cut the peppers in half, remove the stalks, seeds, and white membranes, and cut into large pieces. Cut the tomato crosswise, scald with boiling water and peel off the skin. Halve the skinned tomato, cut out the seeds and finely chop. Peel and finely dice the onion and garlic. Cut the chili pepper in half. Remove the stem and seeds and finely chop.
3. Preheat the oven to 400°F.
4. Heat the olive oil in a large skillet and brown the chicken thighs on all sides until golden brown. Place in an ovenproof dish. Set aside.
5. To the hot skillet, add the onions and garlic and sauté over medium-high heat for 2-3 minutes. Add the remaining paprika and the freshly crushed coriander seeds and cook for 1 minute. Add the chopped bell and chili peppers and chopped chili and sauté for about 5 minutes, until the peppers begin to soften a bit. Then add the tomatoes, date syrup, white wine, and chicken stock and bring to a boil. Remove from heat. Pour sauce over the chicken thighs and spread evenly. Place in oven and bake for 45 minutes. Remove from oven and season with salt and freshly ground pepper.

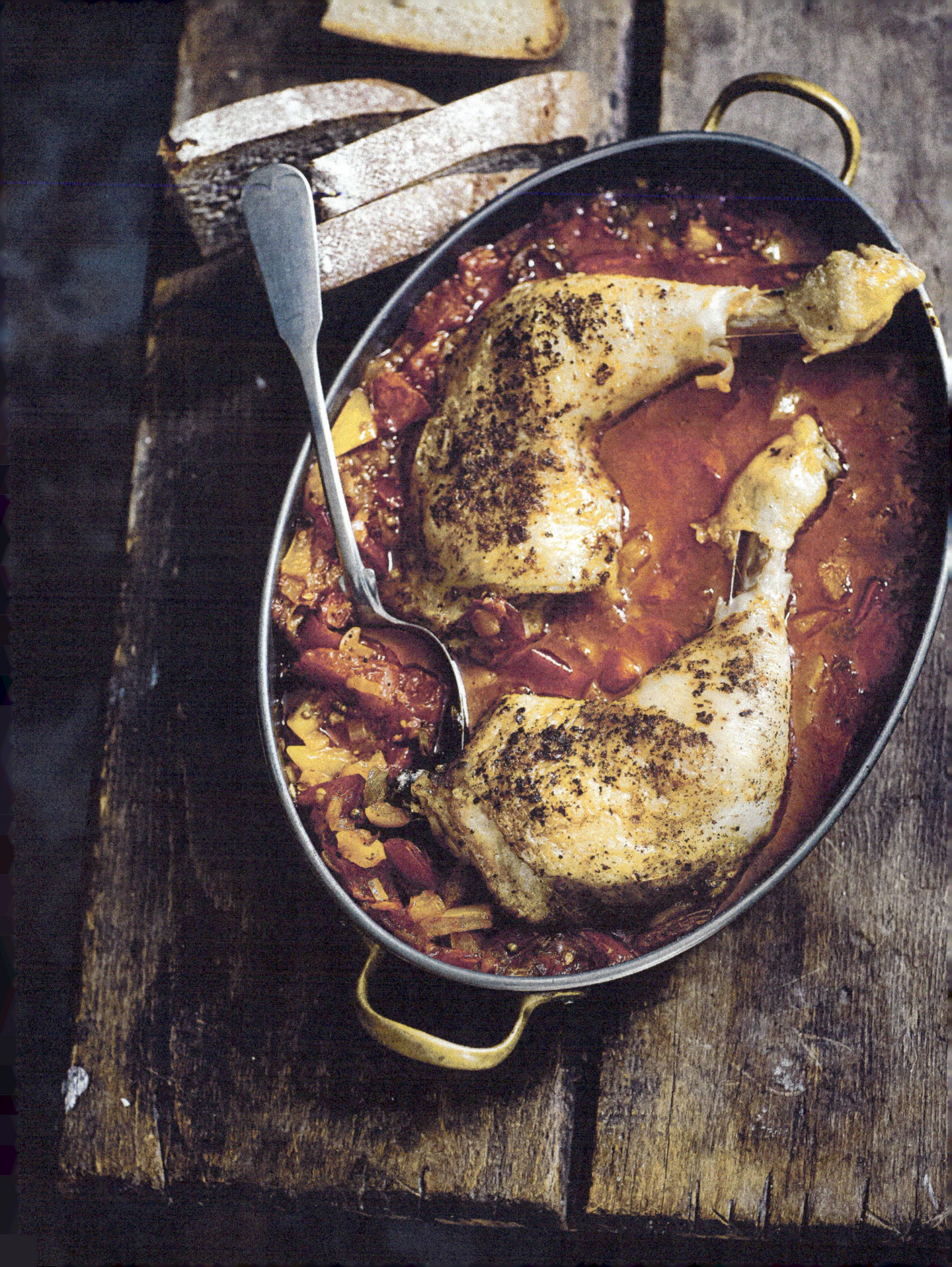

PETCHAH
—CALVES' JELLY WITH EGG

MAKES 10 JELLY MINI-TARTS
PREPARATION: 40 MIN.
COOKING TIME: 3-4 HRS.
JELLYING TIME: 4 HRS.

CALVES' FEET STOCK
2 calves' feet, each cut into 3 pieces
5-6 medium (200 g) carrots
½ lb (200 g) celeriac
2 cloves of garlic
1 onion
10 ½ oz (300 g) beef brisket
1 bay leaf
1 clove
4 black peppercorns
1 pinch of salt

CALVES' FEET JELLY
2 eggs
5 cups (1.2 L) reduced calves' foot stock (see "calves' feet stock" above)
1 medium carrot, diced
1 medium stalk celery, chopped into large chunks
5 chive stems
Cooked beef brisket
Plenty of ice water
Salt
Freshly ground black pepper

TO SERVE
Petchah goes well with bread and a green salad tossed with a tarragon vinaigrette.

CALVES' FEET STOCK

Wash the calves' feet, add to a large pot of water, bring to a boil, and then immediately remove from heat. Drain and rinse the calves' feet. Clean the pot, return the calves' feet, and add about 10 cups of cold water or just enough to cover them. Bring everything to a slow boil, skimming off any foam on the surface.

In the meantime, clean and peel the carrots. Finely dice 1 carrot. Chop the rest into big chunks. Clean and peel the celeriac and chop into big chunks. Take a couple of the large chunks of celeriac and finely dice to create about ½ cup. Set the diced carrot and celeriac aside for the calves' feet jelly preparation below. Add the big chunks of carrot, celeriac, and garlic to the large pot with the calves' feet. Peel and cut the onion in half and roast it in a dry skillet until very dark and add to the pot. Finally, add the brisket, bay leaf, clove, peppercorns and 1 small pinch of salt and simmer everything on low heat for about 3 hours until the brisket is nice and tender. Remove from heat, let cool a bit with the meat in the pot. Remove the meat and strain the stock into a pot through a damp straining cloth. Bring the strained stock to a boil and reduce to 5 cups for use in preparing the calves' feet jelly below.

CALVES' FEET JELLY

1. In the meantime, hard-boil the eggs for 9 minutes, rinse and peel. To the boiling, reduced stock, add the diced carrots and celeriac that you had set aside earlier. Boil for 2 minutes, remove from the stock and rinse under cold water. Wash the chives, pat dry and finely chop. In a large bowl, mix the chives with the diced vegetables. Finely dice the beef brisket, add to the bowl, and mix with the vegetables. Using a knife or egg slicer, cut the eggs into even slices.
2. Season the stock well with salt and freshly ground pepper. Fill a large bowl or sink with ice water, place the pot with the stock in it and allow to cool down. As the stock cools, stir until the collagen from the bone begins to gel.
3. As it begins to jellify, quickly fill 10 ramekins (1/2 cup each) with 1 tablespoon of stock and place 1 egg slice in each. Add the diced vegetables, the beef brisket, and the chives to the remaining stock and quickly fill the ramekins. Place the ramekins in the refrigerator for at least 4 hours until the calves' feet jelly has set.

TO SERVE

Turn the jelly tartlets out of the ramekins and arrange on plates. Serve with bread and a green salad tossed with tarragon vinaigrette.

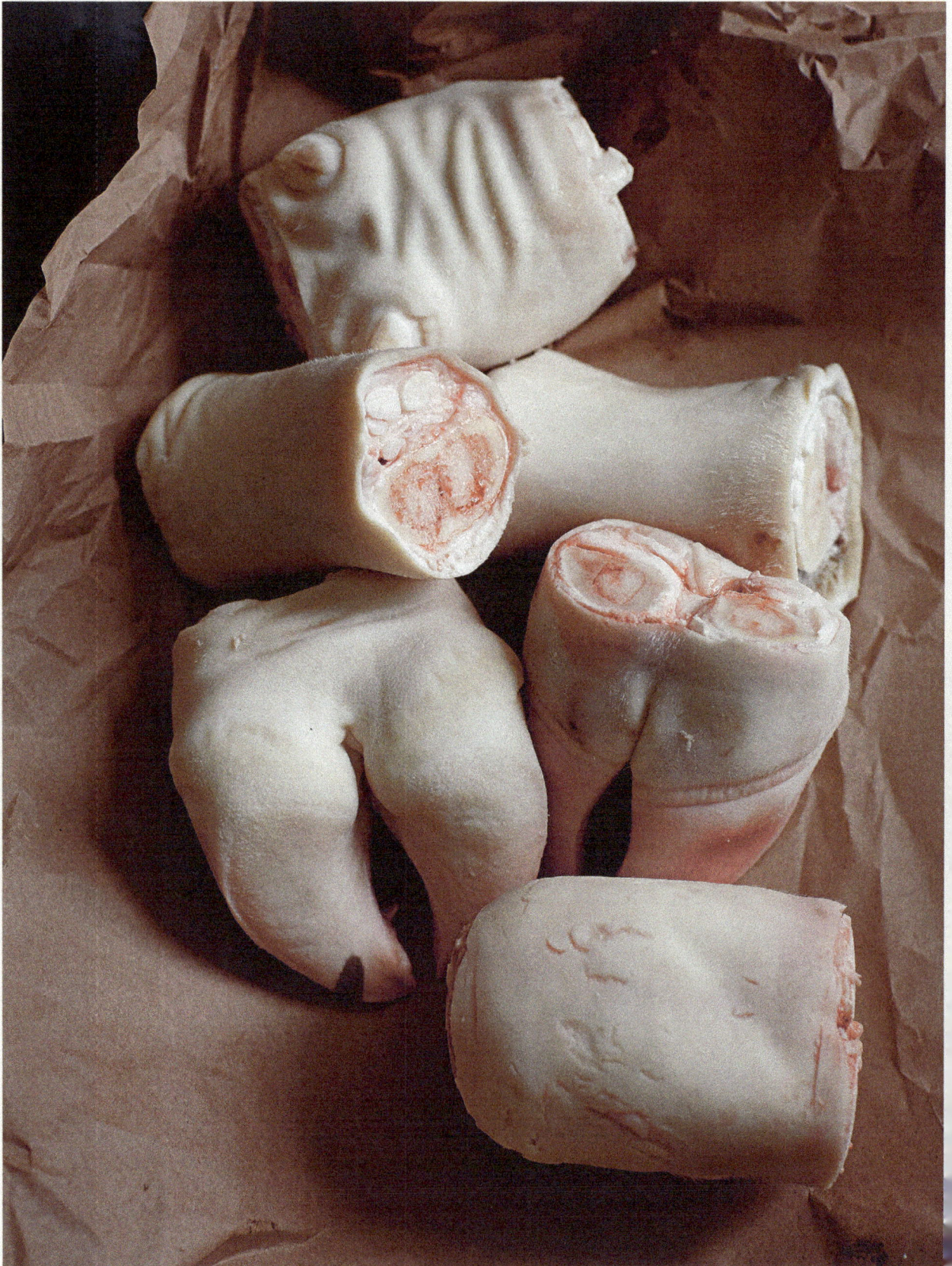

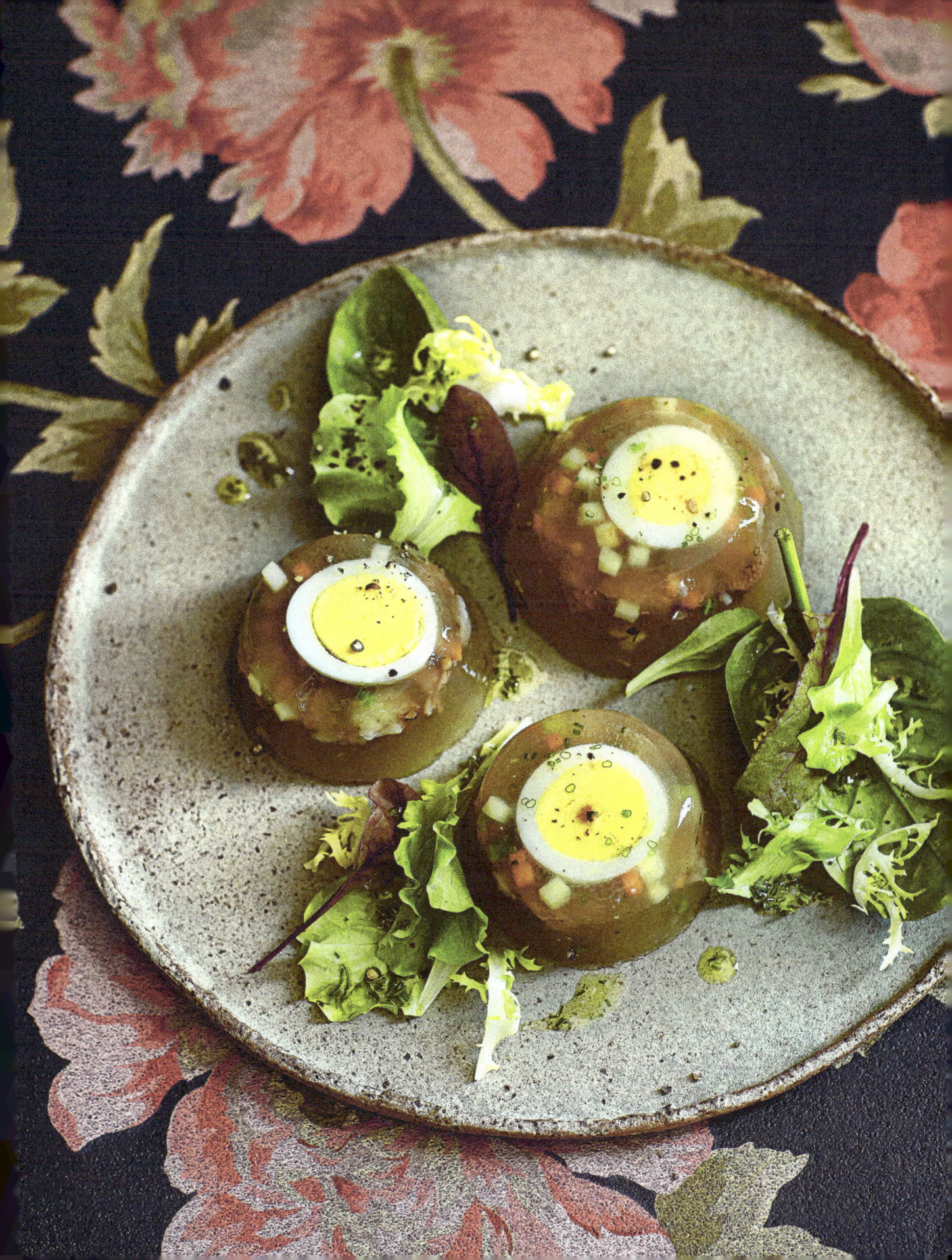

ITAY NOVIK, Berlin

CULINARY TOUR GUIDE AND FOOD STYLIST

Itay Novik is a food stylist and entrepreneur. An Israeli with a strong Italian influence. His goal is to reconnect people with their food and draw more attention to traditional cooking methods.

Itay was born in Tel Aviv, his family has German and Polish roots. When he was a kid, his family only ate Ashkenazi food on holidays. Although his paternal grandmother was not really known for her cooking skills, there was one dish that the whole family loved: schnitzel. Not even Itay's mother could make schnitzel as good as his grandmother. His grandmother also prepared really tasty kreplach dumplings, which she served with chopped chicken liver every year on Yom Kippur.

Schnitzel and kreplach dumplings aside, food was not necessarily a priority in his family. A few years ago, Itay was talking to his mother about his work with food and she joked that she didn't know where his talent in the kitchen came from. Maybe he was born with it? One of his earliest memories is bound up with food. It took place during a family gathering to celebrate the birth of his cousin. He cannot recall all the details, except that he was sitting on the floor in someone's apartment with a swirl of activity around him and experiencing for the first time the smoky flavor and slightly chewy texture of turkey pastrami.

In addition to his early appreciation for food, from a young age he was also already cooking. Both of his parents worked full time, so he had to learn his way around the kitchen to make sure he and his sister had something hot to eat. By age six he already knew how to reheat leftovers and before long he was making up his own dishes. Itay was also a precocious culinary entrepreneur. By age 13, he was baking his own challah and selling it to the neighbors.

Although food always played an important part in his life, he did not pursue it professionally. Instead, in his twenties, he moved to Milan to study industrial design.

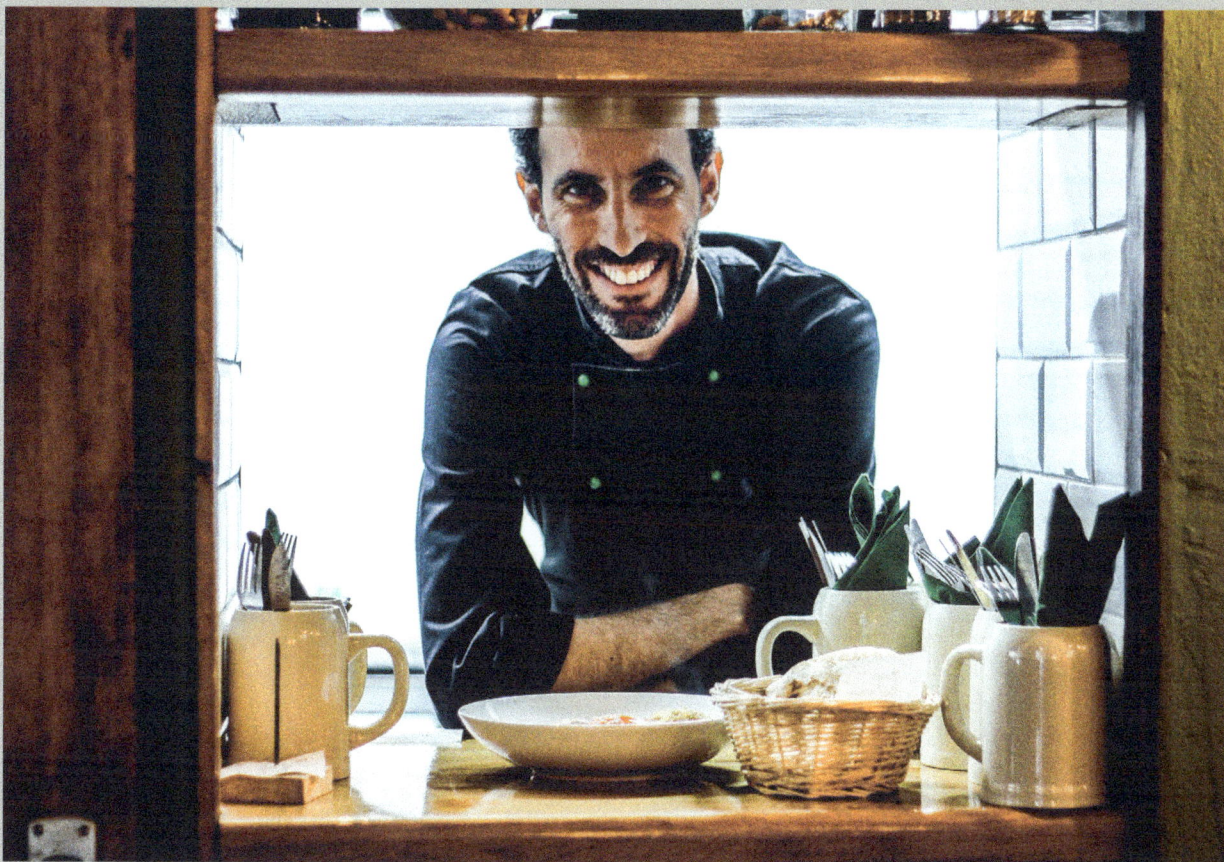

Israeli-born Itay Novik worked as an industrial designer in Milan before starting his own culinary project in Berlin.

After graduation he worked for El-Al airline, which eventually transferred him to Berlin. He quickly fell in love with the city and was determined to stay. In Berlin, he also decided to reinvent himself, to find a way to channel his early passion for food into something remunerative. He started looking for work in the restaurant industry but quickly realized that since he lacked formal training that no one would ever hire him. Plus, he didn't think the job of a classically trained chef would suit him. He'd probably get bored with the strictures and routine. So he decided to create his own dream job. In 2015, he founded "Elements of Food" with the express goal of "reconnecting people to their food." It started with culinary tours and an Israeli pop-up restaurant. People, he realized, were actually willing to spend money on his food. He then expanded his freelance work to include food styling, cooking classes, and events.

Itay counts himself among the fortunate one percent of the population who love what they do and he maintains a sense of adventure and curiosity about food and cooking. Lately, he's been exploring the world of beets; the vegetable fascinates him. Often in Jewish cooking, beets are cooked inattentively, just boiled in water. In addition to trying, with mixed success, to grow them himself, he also experiments with different ways to prepare them, such as one of the recipes featured here in which he turns it into a sorbet to accompany gefilte fish.

Although he cooks a lot of traditional Jewish food, he nonetheless thinks it's important to keep it modern and creative. His kreplach are stuffed with onion confit instead of plain fried onions. He loves chicken soup but doesn't like the chicken in the soup. So after preparing the broth, he removes the chicken and uses it as the filling for kreplach. Working this way, one recipe follows another and Itay expands his repertoire and does his part to keep Jewish cuisine modern and meaningful.

GEFILTE FISH REIMAGINED

SERVES 4
PREPARATION: 2 ½ HRS.
FREEZING TIME FOR THE
   SORBET: 20-30 MIN.
MARINATING TIME
   (CARROTS): 1-2 DAYS

CARROT SALAD
1 teaspoon coriander seeds
3 medium carrots
½ tsp salt
1 cup water

FISH BALLS
7 oz (400 g) cod or skrei filet,
   with or without skin
1 carrot
1 white onion
1 egg
¾ cup (90 g) breadcrumbs
1 tablespoon vegetable oil
1 tablespoon sugar
Salt
Freshly ground white
   pepper

FISH STOCK
1 lb (500 g) white fish fillets, skinned and cut into
   chunks
2 stalks of celery
½ leek, white part only
1 carrot
1 onion
Salt
5-6 black peppercorns

CARROT SALAD

In a dry skillet, toast coriander seeds until they start to smell fragrant. Wash and peel the outer layer from the carrots, then peel lengthwise into long thin strips. Put the carrot strips in a canning jar and sprinkle the roasted coriander seeds on top. Dissolve the salt in the water and pour it into the jar, covering the carrots. Add a little more water, as needed. Close the jar and let the carrots marinate in the refrigerator for 1-2 days.

FISH BALLS

Clean, bone, and coarsely chop the fish fillet. Peel and coarsely dice the carrot and onion. Blend the fish and vegetables in a food processor to create a fine paste. Put into a bowl. Add the egg, breadcrumbs, vegetable oil, sugar, and 1 generous pinch of salt and freshly ground white pepper. Using your hands, mix until it forms a firm, homogeneous mound. Cover with plastic wrap and put in the refrigerator for 1 hour.

FISH STOCK

1. Wash the fish and put in a large pot. Clean and wash the celery and leek. Peel the carrot and the onion. Cut the vegetables into large chunks and add to the pot with the fish. Add salt and the peppercorns. Cover with cold water and gradually bring to a boil, skimming off any foam that rises to the surface. Reduce heat to low, simmer for 45 minutes. Set aside.
2. Meanwhile, remove the fish-ball mixture from the refrigerator and divide into 12 equal portions of about 2 tablespoons each. With wet hands, shape them into balls. Set aside.
3. Pour the fish stock through a fine-mesh strainer into a bowl, removing and then discarding the vegetables or setting them aside for use in another

RED BEET SORBET
2 red beets
1 green apple
1 lemon
4 ¾ cups (1.12 L) beetroot
    juice
4 tablespoons agave syrup

HORSERADISH CREAM
1 piece fresh horseradish
    root (1 ½-inches long)
½ cup (5 ½ oz / 150 g) crè-
    me fraîche
Salt

TO SERVE
Salt
Freshly ground black
    pepper
2-3 sprigs of fresh dill

recipe. Pour the stock back into the pot, return to
a boil. Carefully add the fish balls to the boiling
stock, reduce the heat and cook for 30 minutes.
Remove the pot from the heat and let the fish balls
cool in the stock to room temperature.

RED BEET SORBET
Peel the beets and the apple and cut them
into large chunks. Peel the lemon with a knife,
completely removing any visible pith or white parts,
chop into chunks, removing any seeds. Put the
beets, apples, lemon, beet root juice, and agave
syrup in a blender and purée to a fine consistency.
Put the mixture in an ice cream maker and freeze
for 20-30 minutes.

Tip: If you don't have an ice cream maker, freeze
the chopped beetroot and apple pieces for about
5 hours. Then blend the frozen cubes with the
remaining ingredients. Store in the freezer until
ready to serve, for a maximum of 60 minutes.

HORSERADISH CREAM
Peel the horseradish, finely grate half and mix with
the crème fraîche. Season with salt to taste.

TO SERVE
Divide the horseradish cream among 4 plates and
spread in a slight curve along the edge of each
plate. Arrange 3 fish balls and some marinated
carrot strips in the center of each plate. Drizzle
everything with some cold fish stock and sprinkle
with salt and freshly ground black pepper. Then
grate the remaining horseradish on top and garnish
with some dill. Finally, place 1 large dollop of red
beet sorbet on each plate and serve immediately.

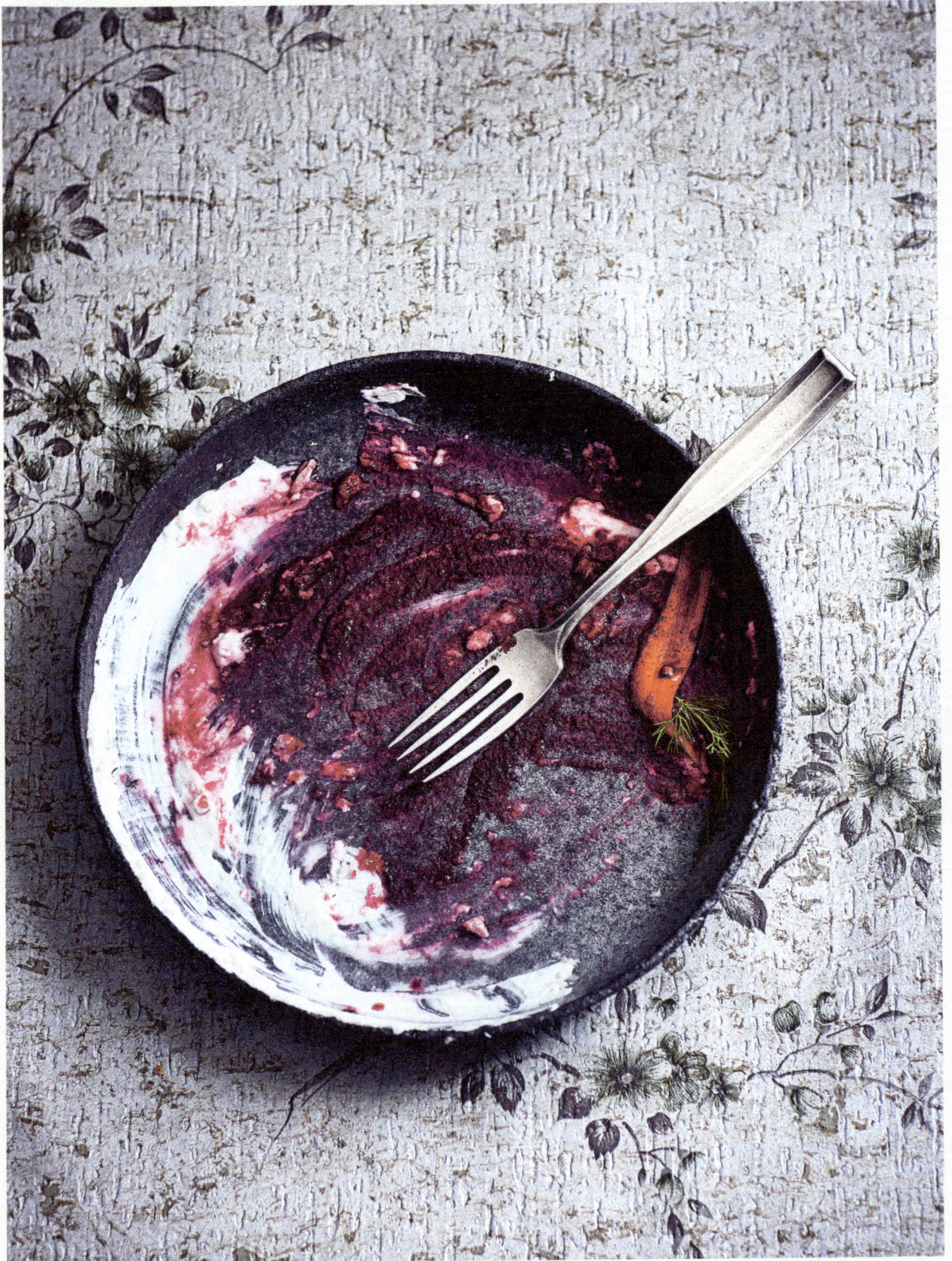

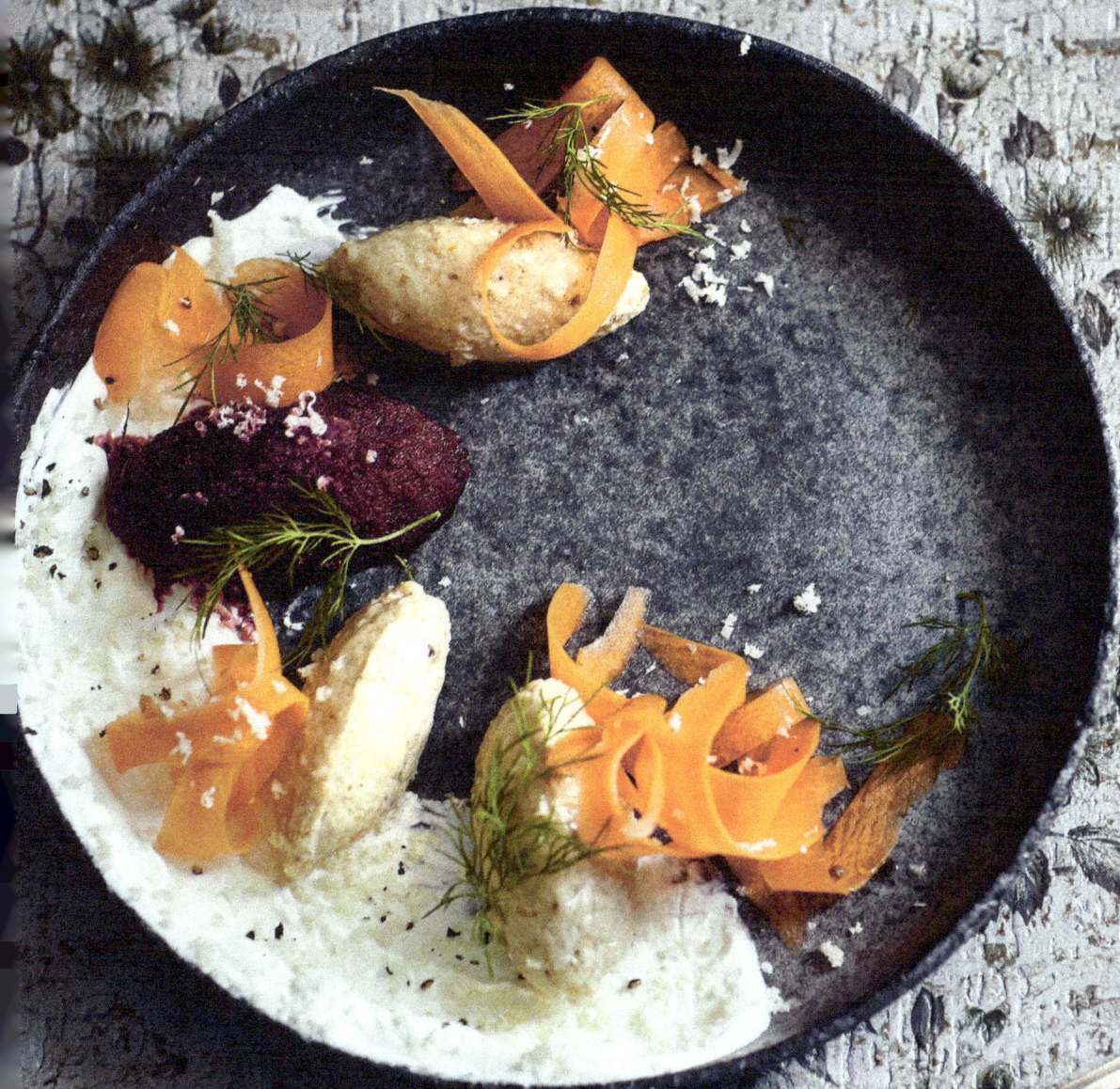

KREPLACH WITH CHICKEN LIVER FILLINGFÜLLUNG

SERVES 2 / MAKES APPROX. 18 PIECES
PREPARATION: 50 MIN.

FILLING
1 medium onion
1 tablespoon vegetable oil
5 ½ oz (150 g) cooked chicken, cut into small
  pieces
5 ½ oz (150 g) fresh chicken liver
Salt
Freshly ground black pepper

FOR STEAMING
2 cups water
1 bay leaf

DOUGH
2 eggs
1 ½ cups boiling water
2 cups (240 g) all-purpose flour
Salt
1 tablespoon vegetable oil
All-purpose flour for work surface

TO SERVE
Sour cream, roasted onions, and pickled beet,
  to taste
Hot chicken stock, to taste

FILLING

1. Finely chop the onion. Heat the vegetable oil in a small saucepan over medium-high heat and sautée the onions until light brown. Add the chicken liver and cook about five minutes, until cooked all the way through. Add the already cooked chicken pieces to the chicken liver-onion mixture and cook for an additional 2 minutes.
2. Remove the pot from the stove. Season with salt and freshly ground pepper, finely chop with a knife and place in a bowl.

DOUGH

1. Separate the eggs and place the whites in one bowl and the yolks in another. In another bowl, mix the boiling water, half of the flour and 1 generous pinch of salt. Whisk together preventing any major lumps from forming. Add the remaining flour, turn out onto a lightly floured work surface, and knead until flour is fully incorporated. Add the egg yolks and vegetable oil one by one and continue to knead until the dough is elastic and easy to shape.
2. Roll out the dough into a ¼-inch thin sheet and using a glass or cup, cut out circles with 3-inch diameters. Place 1 teaspoon of filling in the center of each circle and brush the edges with a little egg white. Fold the dough circles together at three points towards the center, so that you create small, star-shaped pockets.

STEAM

In a saucepan, bring the water to a boil with the bay leaf. Line a steamer with parchment paper, poke small holes in it and place the dumplings on it. Place the steamer insert in the pot with the boiling water, cover with a lid and steam the dumplings for about 6 minutes.

TO SERVE

Serve the steamed dumplings with sour cream, roasted onions, and pickled beet or as a soup accompaniment.

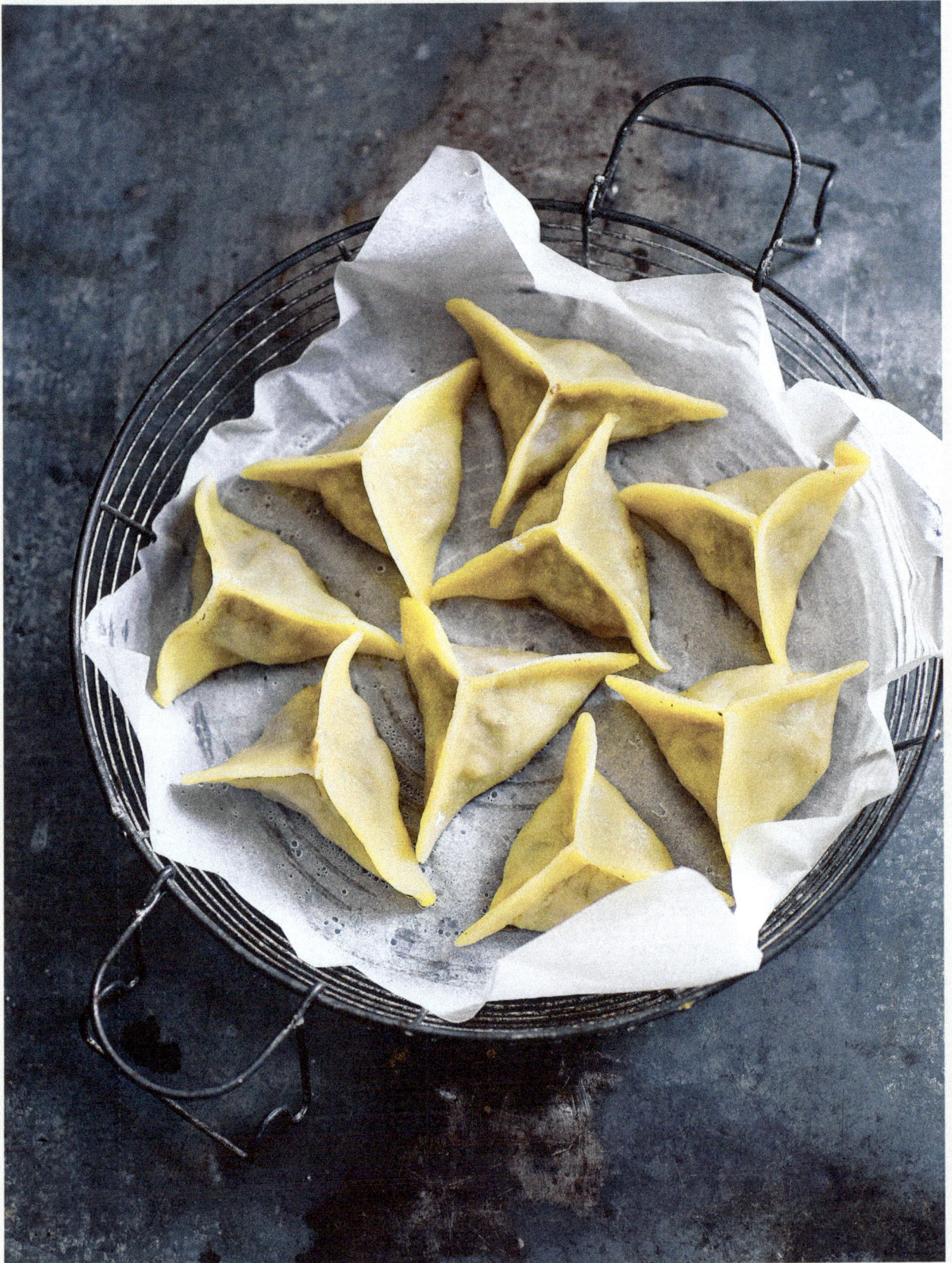

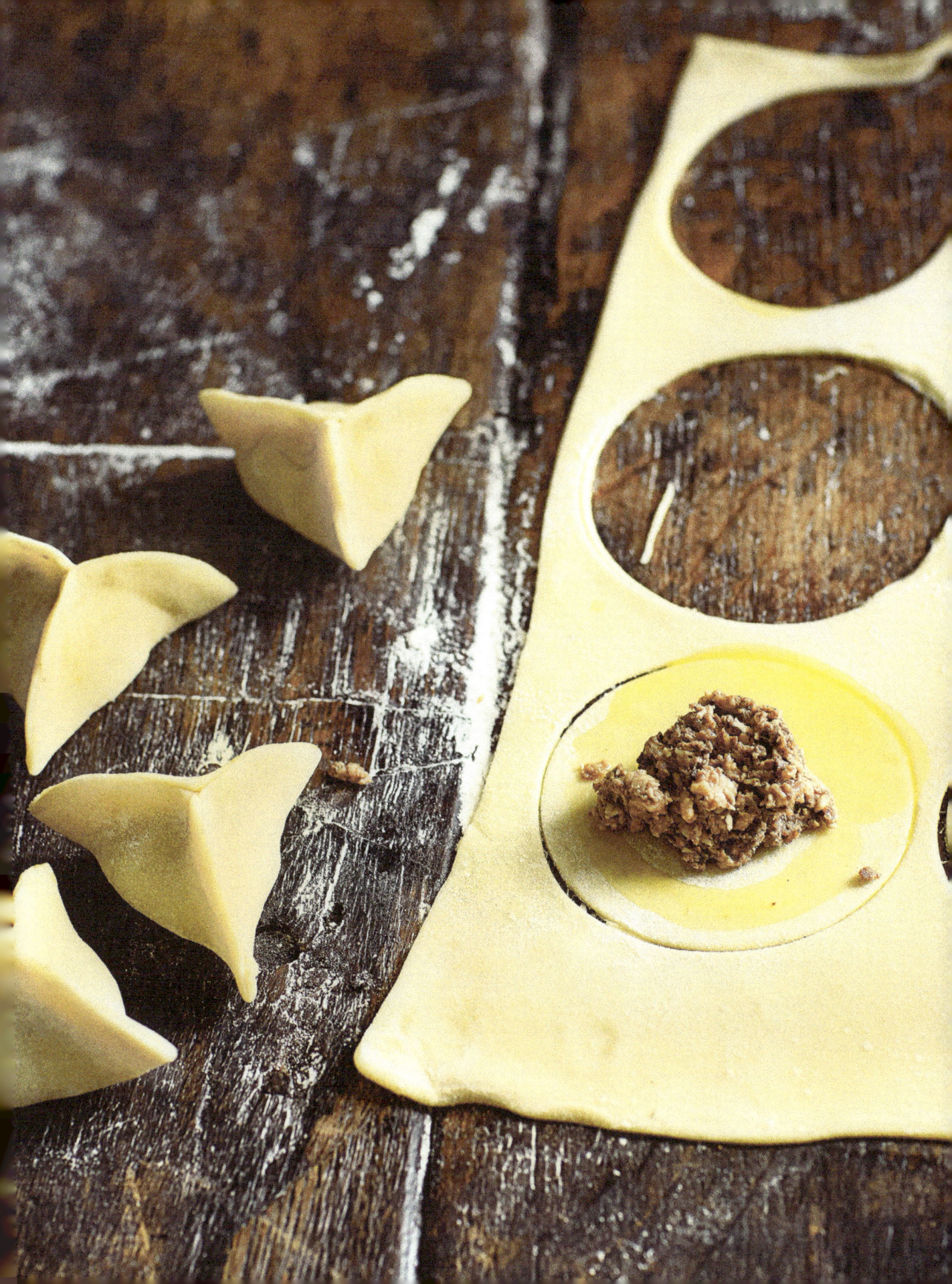

LAUREL KRATOCHVILA, Berlin

IN SEARCH OF THE PERFECT BAGEL

Laurel Kratochvila is single-handedly responsible for bringing good bagels to Berlin. Born in Boston, after meeting her future husband, who was born in the former Czechoslovakia, she moved to Prague where they ran a bookshop together. Although she was settling into her new life ok, she nonetheless missed some elements from home, among them bagels! She searched the city but could not find a proper bagel, prepared the way they were in the US. So she decided to make them herself. Countless attempts and YouTube videos later, she had her bagels, complete with a beautiful crust; exactly the chewy treat she had been looking for. When she and her husband later moved to Berlin

and opened a bookstore, she began selling a few of the bagels at the bookstore. Her baked goods were a hit and the little bookstore had to move to make room for all the bagels. On the bustling Warschauer Straße, they opened up what is now called Fine Bagels and the English-language bookshop, Shakespeare and Sons. Today she supplies half the city with her bagels and in the café you can enjoy a bagel the way it was meant to be—with cream cheese, smoked salmon, and capers.

Food was always at the center of her family's life and plays an important part in her memories of home. When she was young, she cooked with her mother and

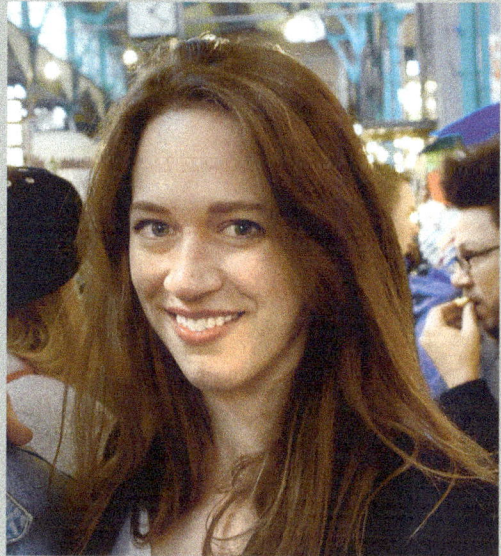

Laurel Kratochvila is known throughout Berlin for her bagels. Born in the United States, she and her husband ran a bookshop together in Prague before moving to Berlin in 2011. From the trendy, family-friendly Berlin neighborhood of Prenzlauer Berg, they moved to the younger, hipper neighborhood of Friedrichshain. On the bustling Warschauer Straße, they opened up what was now called Fine Bagels and the English-language bookshop, Shakespeare and Sons in space that used to house a bookstore that opened in the 1960s.

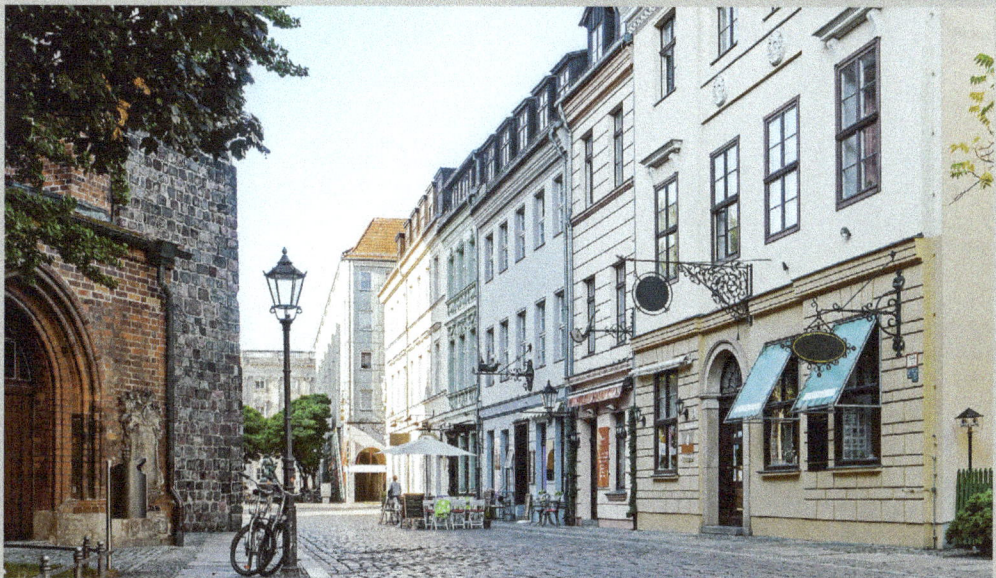

grandmother, whose cooking drew on their Polish-Jewish origins. These early influences continue to shape Laurel's approach to cooking. Not all childhood memories related to food are positive, however. Her first memory of food was somewhat traumatic. At the tender age of six, she nearly choked on some stuffed cabbage. To help cope with the traumatic memory she's become adept at making stuffed cabbage. That's one way to cope with traumatic memories!

Laurel is a savvy entrepreneur and a natural host. In addition to running Fine Bagels, recently she also wrote a cookbook, *New European Baking: 99 Recipes for Breads, Brioches and Pastries*. Although she herself isn't religious, she nonetheless still loves to celebrate the High Holidays by inviting people over either to her home or to the café.

Looking back on her unexpected foray into running a bakery, which has required a lot of work and multi-tasking, she observes how she has now learned to delegate better. This new-found ability to "let go" of some things, entrusting them to others, has made room for more peace to enjoy her daily life. And maybe even a bagel or two now and again.

BAGEL
BASE RECIPE

MAKES 12 BAGELS
PREPARATION: 70 MIN.
RESTING TIME: 11 HRS.
COOKING & BAKING
**   TIME: 20-25 MIN.**

PRE-DOUGH
3 1/3 cups (450 g) all-pur-
    pose flour
2 ¼ teaspoons (7 g) or 1
    packet active dry yeast
2 teaspoons dark malt
    syrup (or dark honey)
1 ½ cups (340 mL) luke-
    warm water

MAIN DOUGH
2 ½ teaspoons salt
1 tablespoon dark malt
    syrup (or dark honey)
2 tablespoons lukewarm
    water
1 cup (110 g) all-purpose
    flour
Pre-dough yeast (see "pre-
    dough" above)
1 tablespoon neutral
    vegetable oil to grease
    the bowl

FINAL STEPS
All-purpose flour for the
    work surface
Fine wheat semolina for
    work surface
Soaked, dried onions,
    poppy seeds or sesame
    seeds for sprinkling, as
    desired

PRE-DOUGH

1. Mix the flour and the dry yeast in a bowl. Dissolve the malt syrup in the lukewarm water, add it to the flour and mix first with a wooden spoon and then, using your hands, on a lightly floured surface knead it into a dough. (Note: the pre-dough will be a bit dry and brittle at first.)
2. Cover the bowl with plastic wrap or a kitchen towel and let rise in a warm place for 2 hours or until double in size.

MAIN DOUGH

1. Dissolve the salt and malt syrup in the water and add to the pre-dough together with additional flour. Using your hands, knead until a silky, homogeneous dough is formed. (Note: some perseverance is needed here; this will take about 5-7 minutes. Using a food processor is not advisable, as the dough is so firm that it could damage the food processor).
2. Finally, place the dough in a lightly oiled bowl, cover and let rise in the refrigerator overnight or about 8 hours.

FINAL STEPS

1. Preheat 2 pizza stones or 2 baking sheets in the oven to 375°F.
2. Remove the dough from the bowl and divide into 12 equal portions. Lightly dust a large wooden board with a little flour. With the slightly sticky side down, use the hollow of your hand to turn each portion of dough into balls. Work in a circular motion, applying gentle pressure, until the top of the dough is closed and slightly stretched.
3. Cover the balls and let rise for 30 minutes.

4. Using both of your hands, flatten 1 dough ball at a time and using both thumbs, press a hole through the center. Pull the resulting ring apart a little in circular motions so that a 2-inch hole and the shape of a bagel is formed. Sprinkle a baking sheet with wheat semolina and place the bagels on it, cover and let rise for another 30 minutes.

5. In a large pot, bring water to a boil, then reduce to a simmer. Now, in stages, slide 4-6 bagels into the simmering water and cook each side for 1 minute. (Note: the dough's consistency is just right if the dough pieces float to the surface immediately. Otherwise, before turning them over, wait for the moment until they do rise to the surface).

6. Place the boiled pieces of dough on 2 baking sheets lined with parchment paper, leaving plenty of space between them. Immediately sprinkle with soaked, dried onions, poppy seeds or sesame seeds, as desired.

7. Carefully set the boiled dough onto either the preheated hot pizza stone or baking sheets. Bake for 15-20 minutes until golden brown. Allow to cool.

Tip: Since the preparation of the bagels is relatively time-consuming and involved, it is worth making the double recipe right away. You can freeze the extras; they will taste almost as good as the fresh ones. If you like to experiment, you can use half rye flour or spelt flour and/or mix into the dough herbs and spices like caraway or coriander seeds.

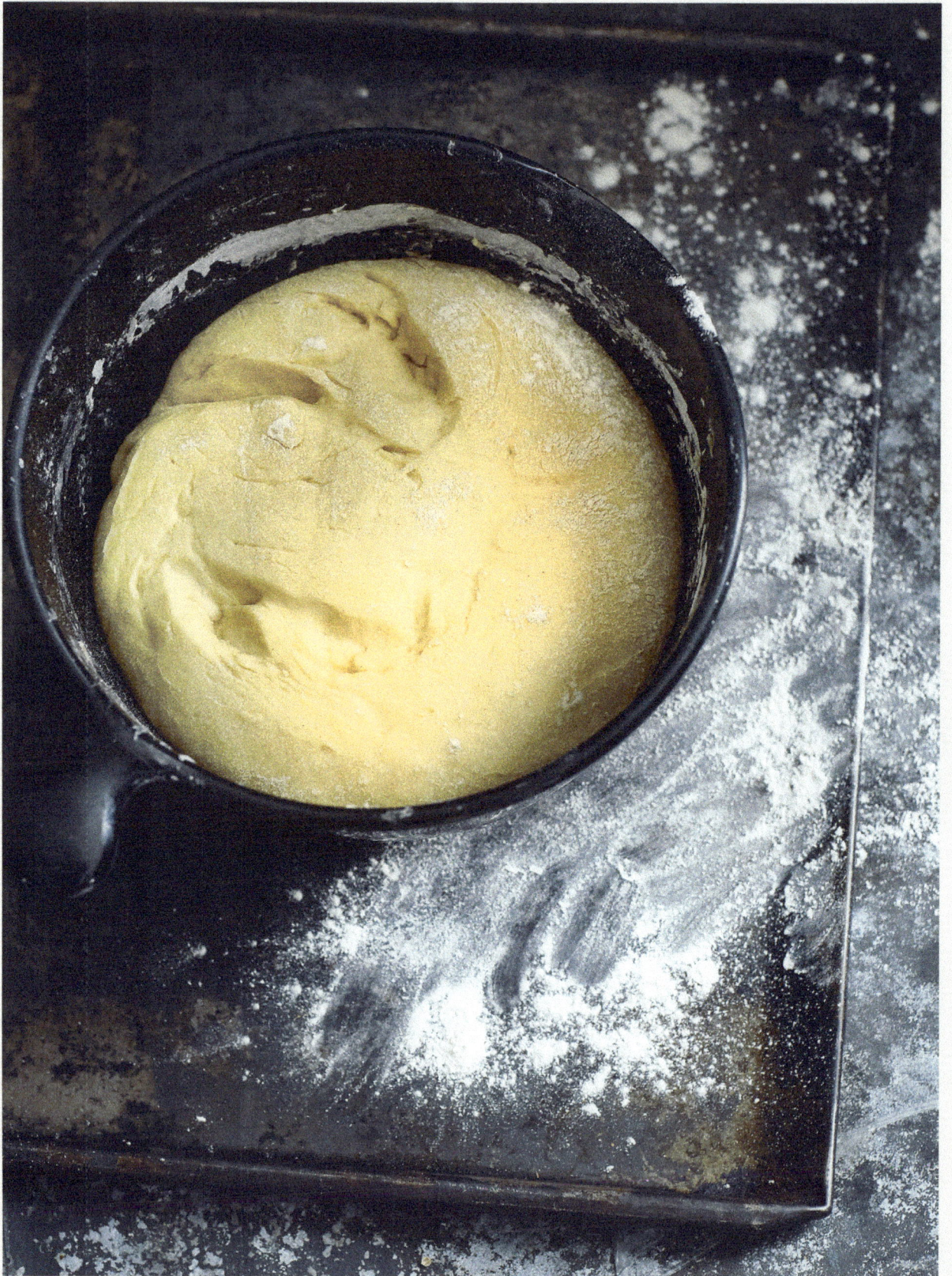

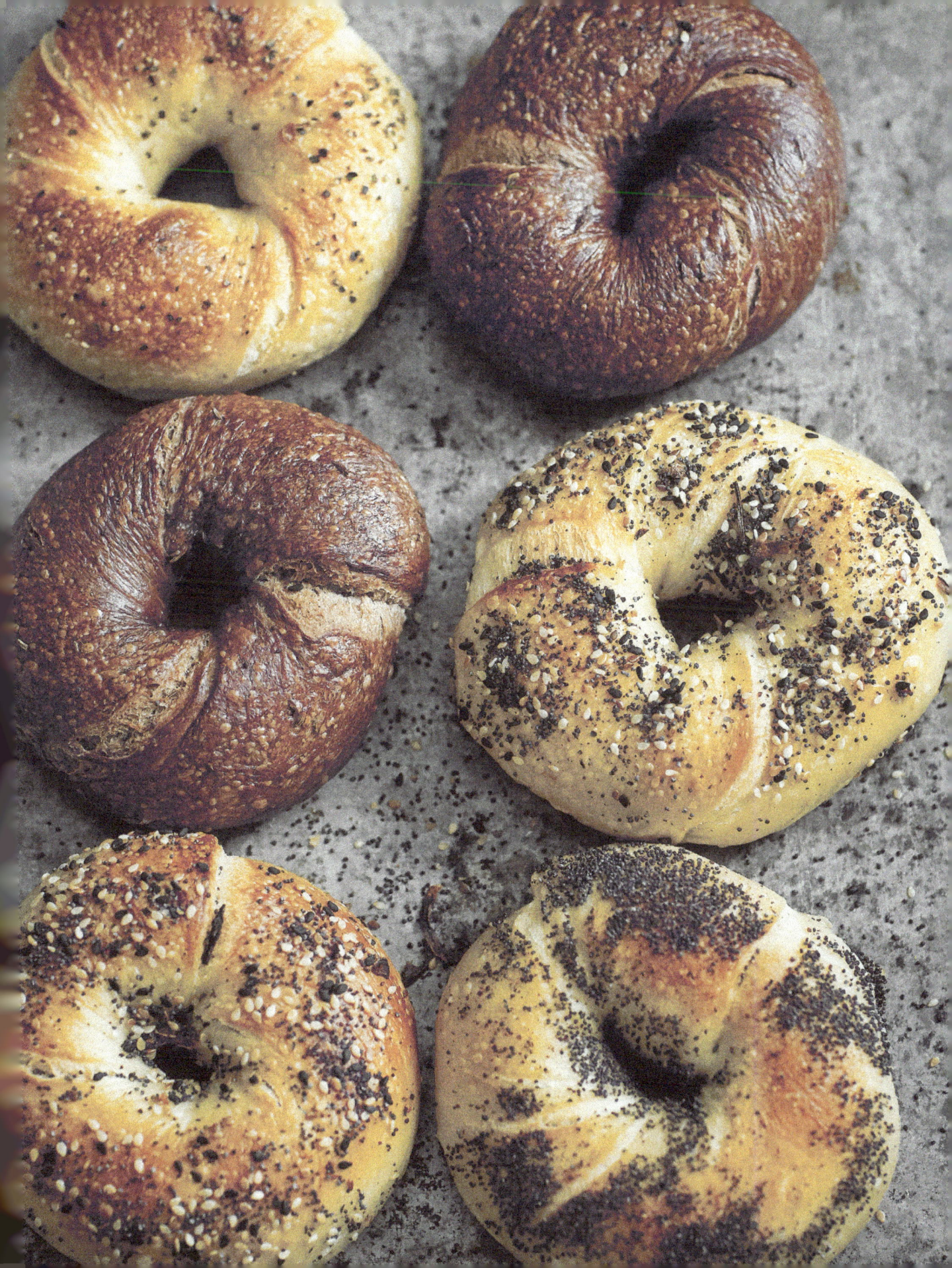

BAGELS
THREE WAYS

MAKES 2 BAGELS EACH
PREPARATION: 10- 15 MIN. PER TYPE OF BAGEL

ONION BAGEL WITH AVOCADO,
HUMMUS & RED BEET
2 onion bagels
1 ripe avocado
¼ cup (50 g) Greek yogurt
2 tablespoons tahini
1 organic lemon
1 teaspoon lemon zest
Salt
Freshly ground black pepper
½ cup (50 g) walnuts
1 beet
Handful (10 g) of cilantro
1 tablespoon roasted sesame oil
2 teaspoons za'atar

POPPYSEED BAGEL WITH
HORSERADISH,CREAM CHEESE, SMOKED
SALMON & CAVIAR
2 poppy seed bagels
¾-inch fresh horseradish root
½ cup (100 g) cream cheese
1 handful of baby spinach
4 ½ oz (120 g) smoked salmon
1 ¾ oz (50 g) trout caviar

RYE BAGEL WITH PASTRAMI BBQ &
MARINATED ONIONS
2 rye bagels
2 small red onions
1 tablespoon white wine vinegar
1 tablespoon agave syrup
Coarse sea salt
Freshly ground black pepper
1 beef tomato
2 teaspoons mayonnaise
2 teaspoons smoky BBQ sauce
4 ½ oz (120 g) pastrami
2 teaspoons zhug (see recipe p. 22)

ONION BAGEL WITH AVOCADO-HUMMUS & RED BEET

Cut the avocado in half and scoop out the pit. Remove the avocado flesh from the skin with a spoon, place in a bowl and mash with a fork. Stir in the yogurt and tahini and season with 1 squeeze of a lemon, salt and pepper. In a dry skillet, toast the walnuts until golden brown, then set aside. Peel the beet and grate coarsely into a bowl. Wash the cilantro, pluck the leaves from the stems, finely chop the stems, and add to the grated beet with half of the leaves. Season the avocado-hummus with 1 tablespoon lemon juice, sesame oil, 1 teaspoon finely grated lemon zest, salt and pepper. Cut the bagels in half, spread the hummus on the bottoms. Top with the beet and cilantro salad, then add the nuts, za'atar, and remaining cilantro. Place the top bagel halves on top.

POPPY SEED BAGEL WITH HORSERADISH, CREAM CHEESE, SMOKED SALMON & CAVIAR

Peel and finely grate the horseradish and mix half with the cream cheese until smooth. Wash the spinach and spin dry thoroughly. Cut the bagels in half. Spread the bottom halves with the horseradish cream cheese mixture. Layer the spinach and salmon on top. Top with the caviar and the remaining freshly grated horseradish.

RYE BAGEL WITH PASTRAMI BBQ & MARINATED ONIONS

Cut the onions in half, peel and cut into thin strips. Place them in a bowl with the vinegar, agave syrup, 1 pinch of salt and pepper and let sit for 10 minutes. Cut the tomato into slices. Cut the bagels in half. Spread the bottom halves with mayonnaise and BBQ sauce. Layer the tomato slices, pastrami, and drained onions and top each with ½ teaspoon zhug.

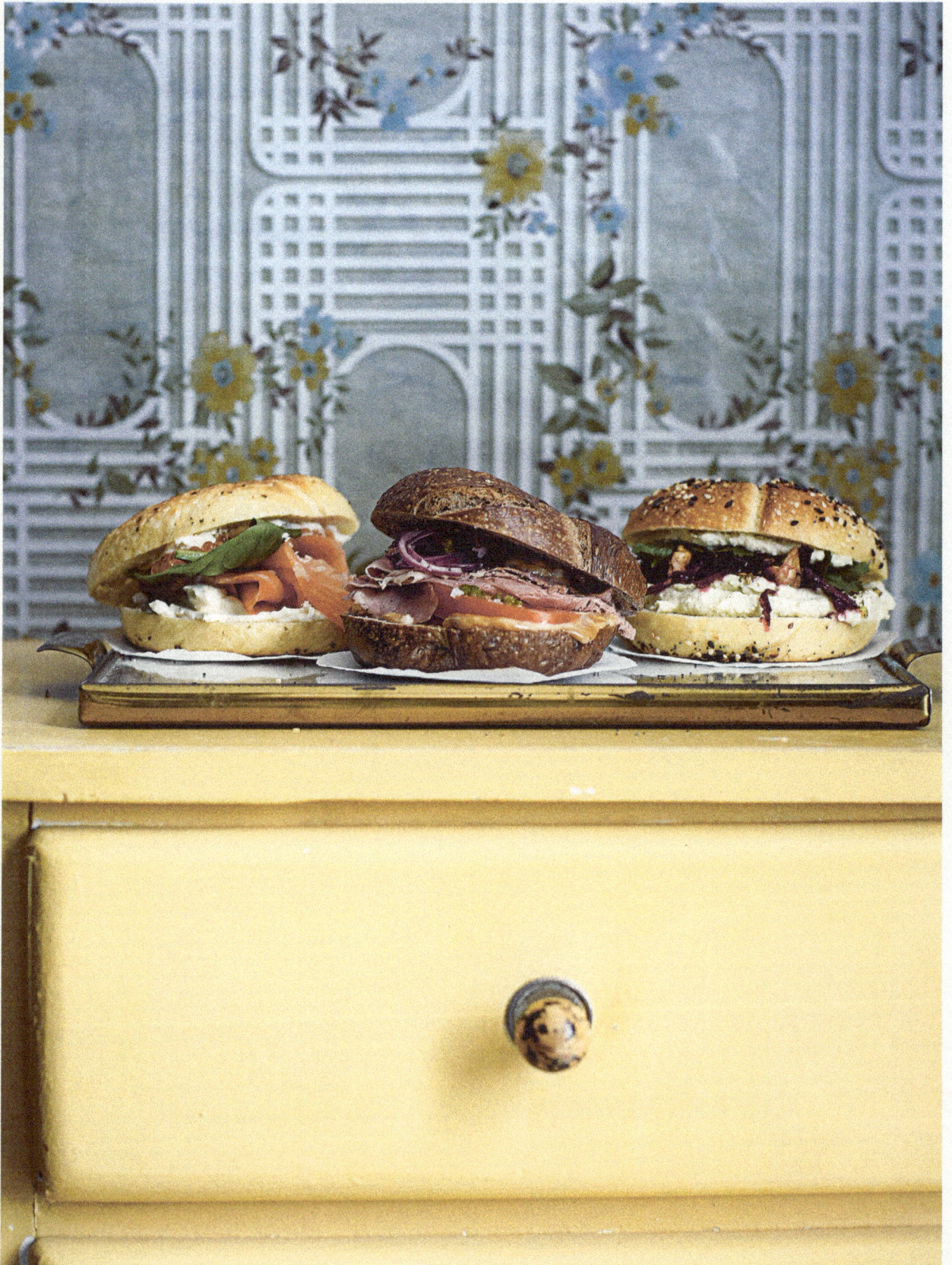

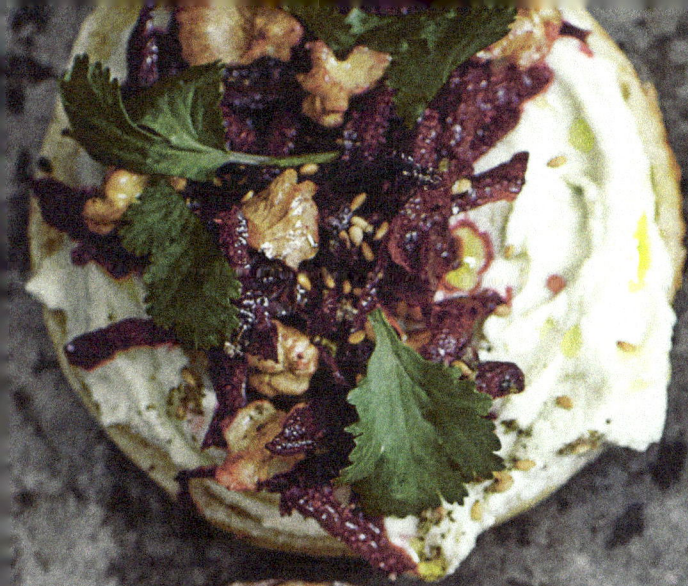

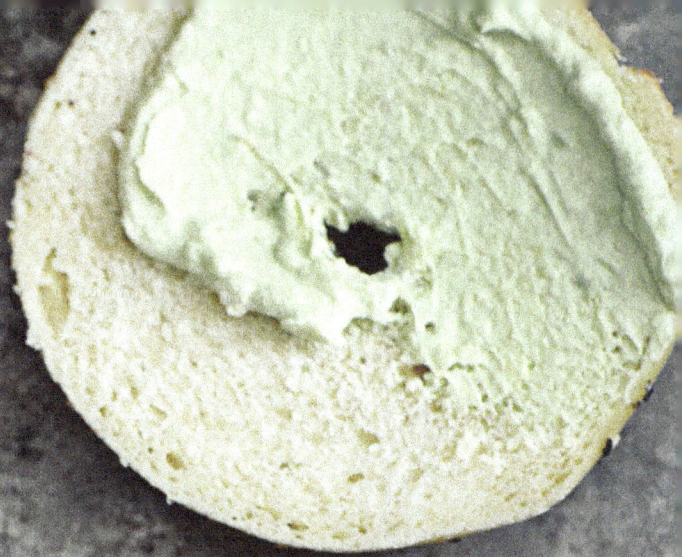

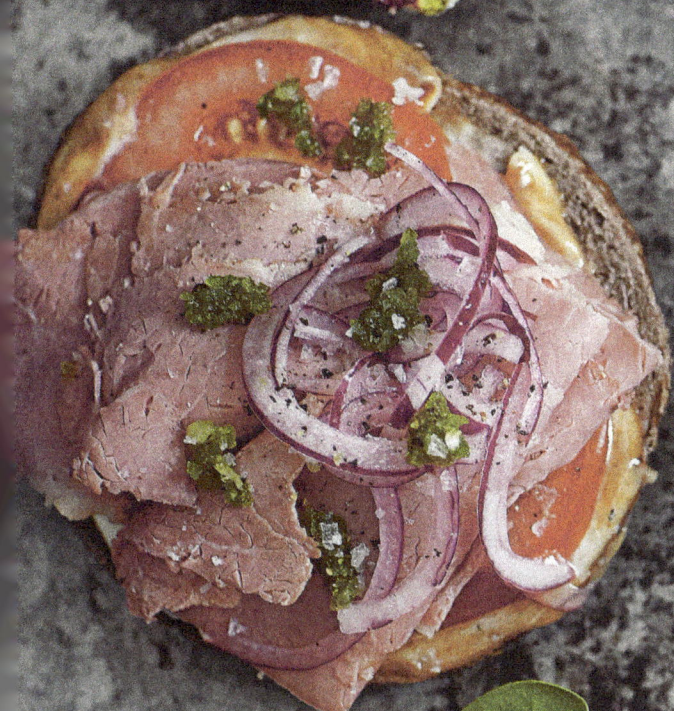

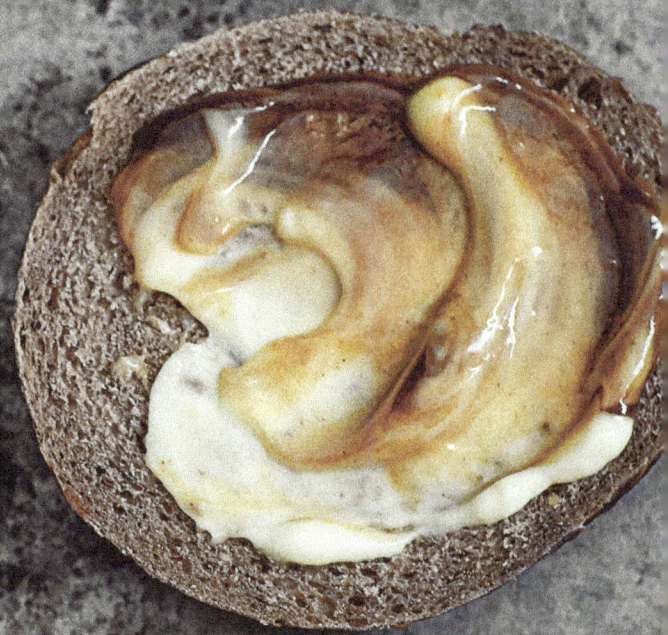

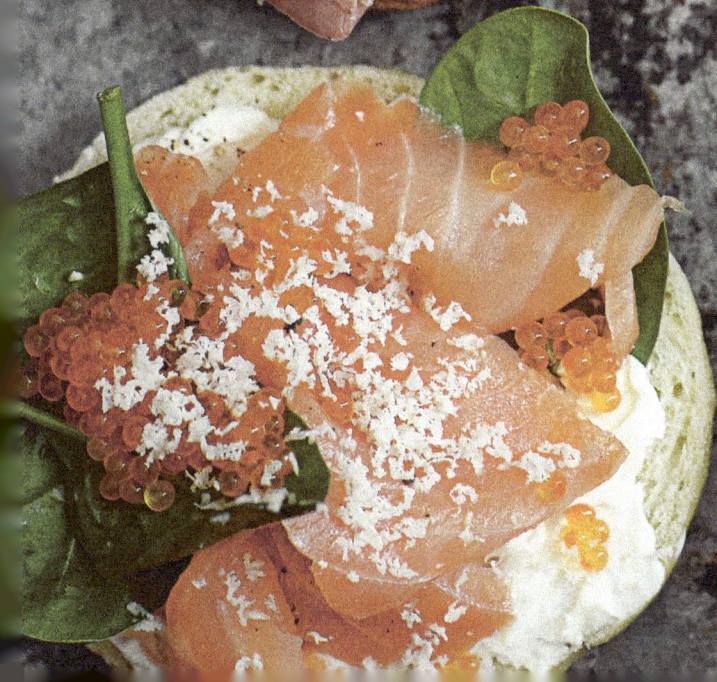

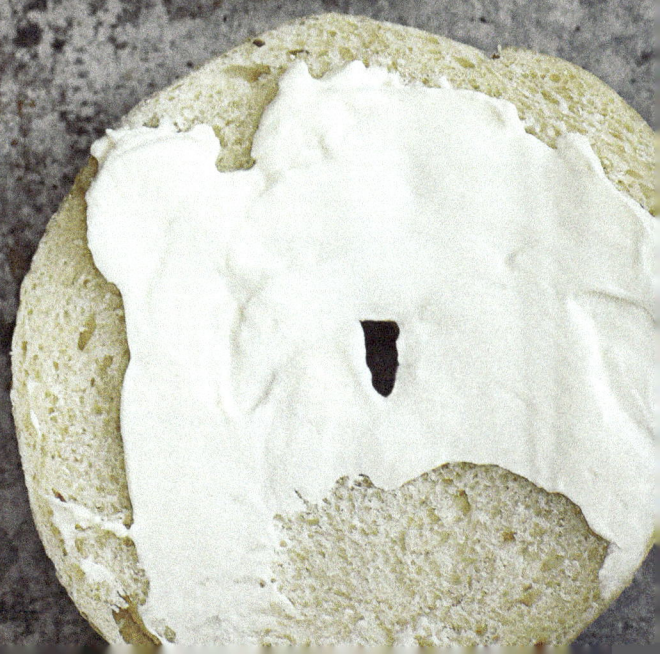

HOLISHKES —STUFFED CABBAGE ROLLS

SERVES 4-6
PREPARATION: 40 MIN.
COOKING TIME: 90 MIN.

CABBAGE ROLLS
1 head fresh white
    cabbage
Salt
2 lb (800 g) ground beef
2 eggs
½ cup (80 g) onion, finely
    chopped
2 teaspoons onion powder
Freshly ground black
    pepper

SAUCE
1, 28 oz (750 g) can diced
    tomatoes
Juice of ½ lemon
¼ cup (60 g) brown sugar
Salt
Freshly ground black
    pepper

TO SERVE
Cooked rice or mashed
    potatoes, to taste

CABBAGE ROLLS

1. Bring a large pot of lightly salted water to a boil. Make a wedge-shaped cut in the stalk of the cabbage and remove it. Cook the cabbage head in the water for about 8 minutes until the leaves have turned a slightly more intense green color. Lift the cabbage out of the water and peel 12 leaves off the cabbage head, one at a time, being sure to keep them whole. Pat the cabbage leaves dry on a kitchen towel. Keep the cooking water and use the remaining cabbage for another recipe.

2. For the filling, put the ground beef, eggs, chopped onions, and onion powder in a bowl. Season with salt and freshly ground pepper and mix everything together. Divide into 6 equal portions. Place 2 cabbage leaves on top of each other, slightly overlapping, spread the filling on the bottom leaf. Fold in the sides and roll the cabbage leaf up and secure with a little kitchen twine, seam side down.

SAUCE

1. Combine the tomatoes, sugar, and lemon juice and season vigorously with salt and freshly ground pepper. If desired, add some cabbage water (approx. ¼-½ cup). This adds some additional flavor and a finer consistency.

2. Spread 2 tablespoons of the sauce in a cast-iron or ovenproof pot. Place the cabbage rolls side by side and pour the remaining sauce over them. Cover the pot with a lid and shake gently so that the sauce is well distributed around each roll. Slowly bring sauce to a boil, reduce heat and simmer for about 1 ½ hours. Finally, season the sauce with salt and pepper to taste.

TO SERVE

Divide the cabbage rolls among plates and remove the kitchen twine. Drizzle with the braising sauce and serve with cooked rice or mashed potatoes, as desired.

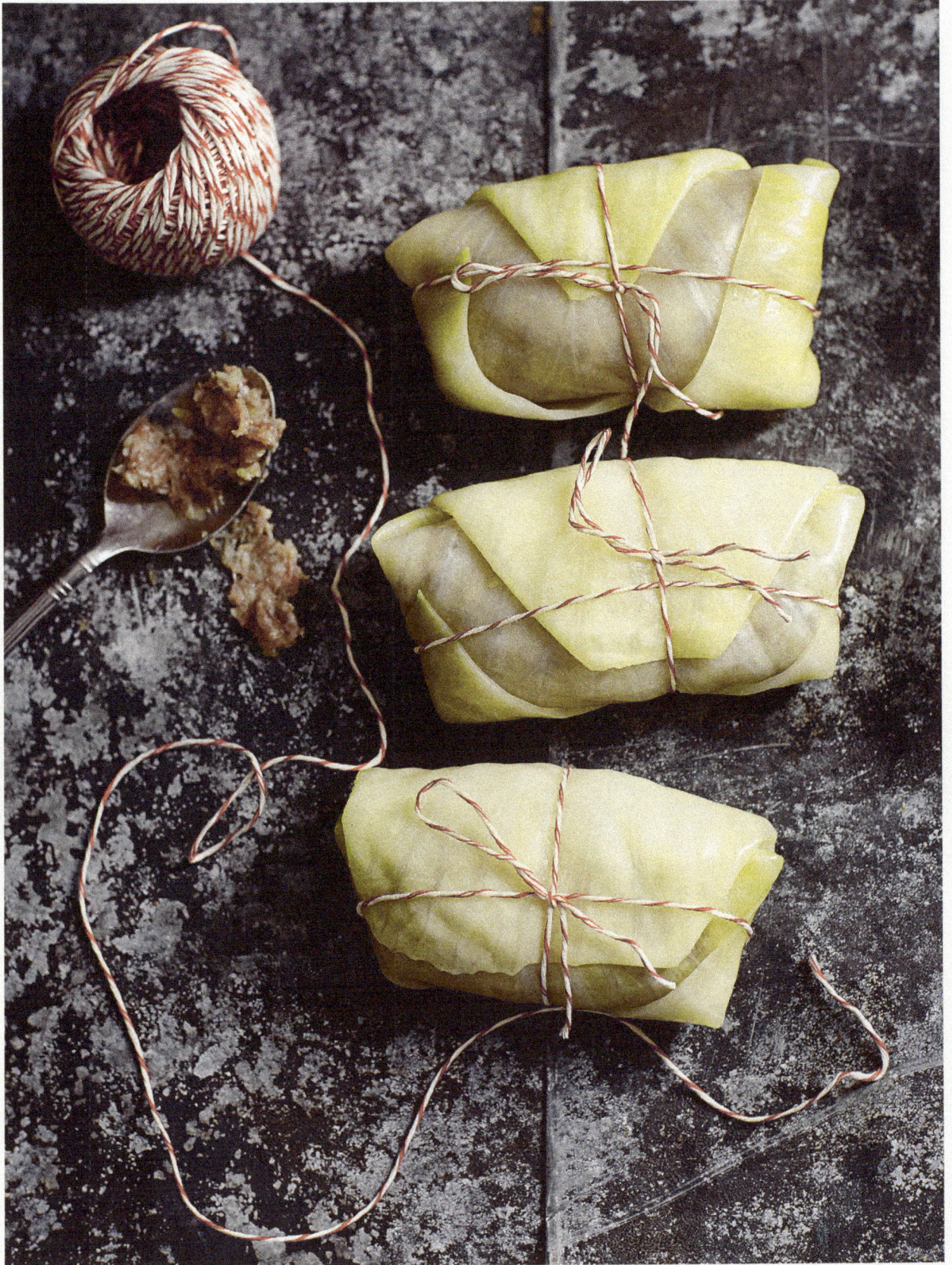

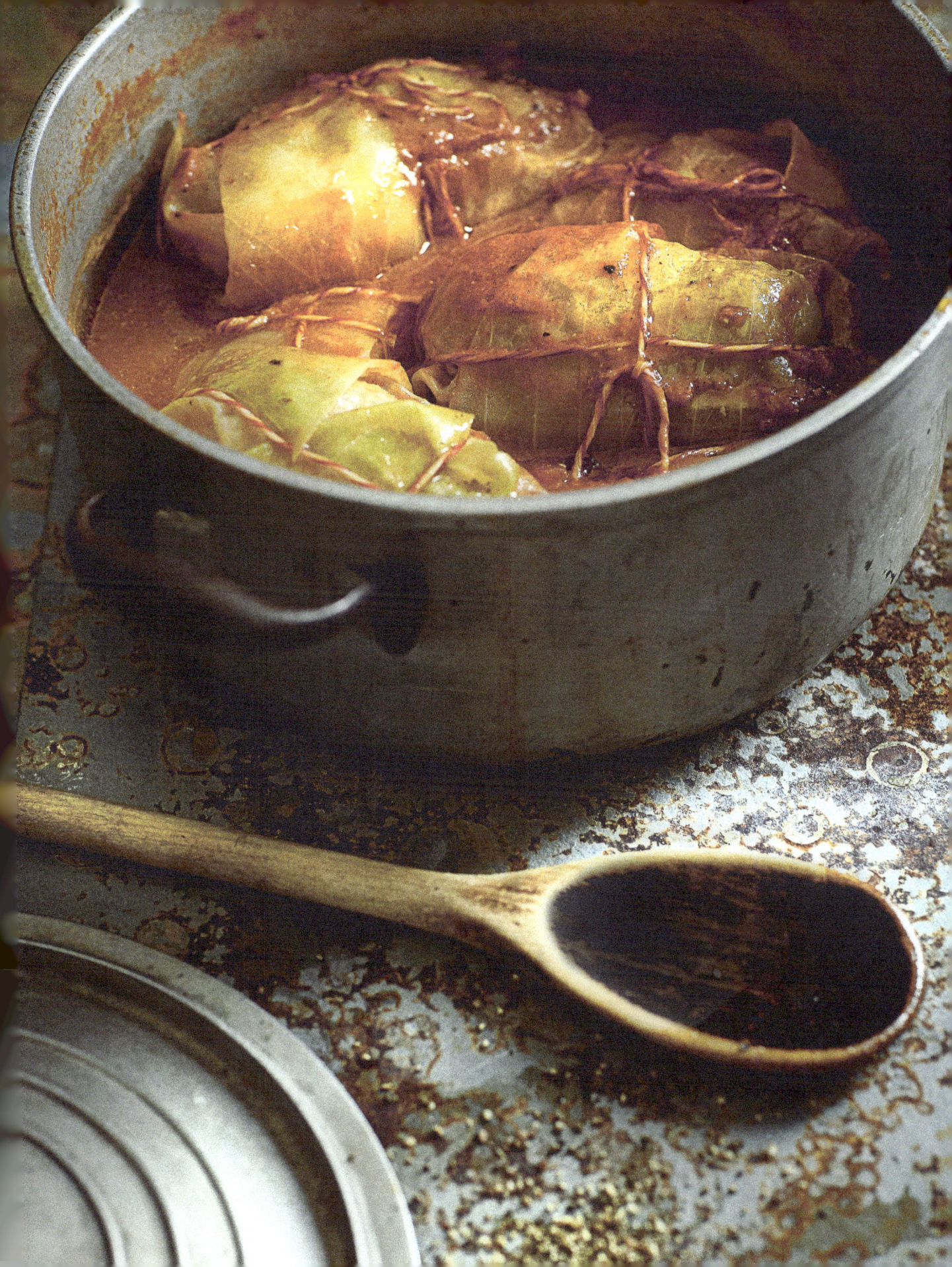

MANDEL BREAD

MAKES ABOUT 50 COOKIES
PREPARATION: 90 MIN.

MANDEL BREAD
6 eggs
2 ¼ cups (450 g) sugar
1 cup (225 mL) neutral
  vegetable oil (such as
  sunflower oil)
¼ cup (55 mL) orange juice
1 teaspoon salt
5 ¾ cups (720 g) cake flour
2 ½ tsp baking powder
1 ¾ cups (200 g) chopped
  almonds
1 cup (200 g) raisins
Cinnamon-sugar for sprinkling

MANDEL BREAD

1. Preheat the oven to 350°F. Line 2 baking sheets with parchment paper.

2. Put the eggs and sugar in a mixing bowl. Using a hand mixer or food processor beat for 4-6 minutes until a whitish fluffy cream is formed. Add in the vegetable oil, orange juice, and salt, and continue beating for 1 minute. In a separate bowl, mix the flour with the baking powder and add to the egg mixture. Quickly mix everything to form a dough. Add the chopped almonds and raisins and knead until a homogeneous dough is formed.

3. Divide the dough into 4 equal portions and form rolls of equal length. Place 2 rolls on each of the baking sheets. Using a rolling pin, gently roll over each piece 1 to 2 times, giving them a more oval, slightly crescent shape. Sprinkle some cinnamon-sugar over them and bake for 25 minutes until light brown.

4. Remove the loaves from the oven and let cool for 5 minutes. Reduce the oven temperature to 200°F. Cut each loaf into ¾-inch-thick slices and lay these side by side on the baking sheet, cut-side down. Sprinkle each slice with cinnamon-sugar and put back in the oven for 40 minutes until they become crunchy in texture. Then sprinkle again with cinnamon-sugar and dry in the oven for 40 minutes.

Tip: Mandel bread will keep for a long time in a sealed tin. A cookie jar is best. They are the perfect accompaniment to a cup of coffee.

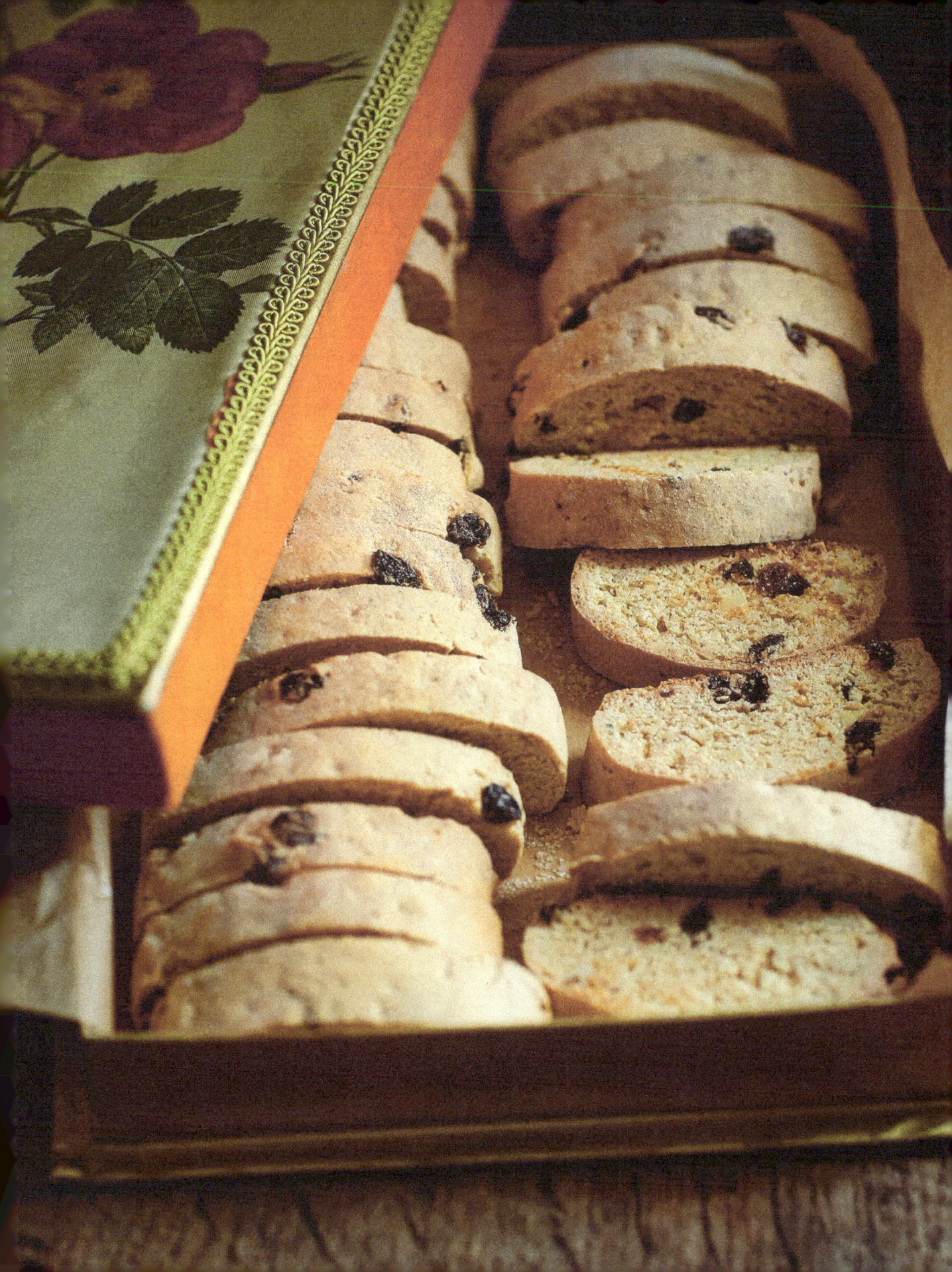

ARIELLE ARTSZTEIN, Berlin

IN LOVE WITH MACARONS

Arielle Artsztein was born with a love for French cooking. The daughter of a Polish father and a North African mother, Arielle grew up in Paris. When she turned twelve, her family moved to Israel. But they always maintained a connection to France and spent every summer in Antibes on the Côtes d'Azur. Her father, whom she describes as a real gourmet, made sure that their travel itinerary revolved around visiting Michelin-starred restaurants. At some point, however, the Michelin-trips became too much for her and she refused to spend her vacation dedicated solely to visiting restaurants. After that they spent only half of their vacation time in high-end restaurants. Even if she grew weary of such fare, they exposed her to the best of French cuisine at a young age. Later she balanced this experience with exposure to more simple but no less impressive French fare, cultivating an appreciation for the fact that a good dish starts with good products.

Beyond those summer vacations in France, her father influenced her relationship to food in other ways. As a native of Poland, he grew up eating typical Eastern European cuisine, which consisted of dishes like cholent and gefilte fish. After they got married, Arielle's mother learned how to prepare such dishes for him and later Arielle too. Whether of French or Jewish origin, food was a charged theme growing up. Like a lot of Holocaust survivors, Arielle's father had a complicated, obsessive relationship with food. Arielle says that in their home, "Food was something burdensome. The pressure to eat was always present." This fraught relationship with food accompanied her into early adulthood.

It wasn't until she completed her military service in the Israeli army that she developed a healthier relationship to eating. The army had a wonderful cook with whom she spent a lot of time and from whom she learned a

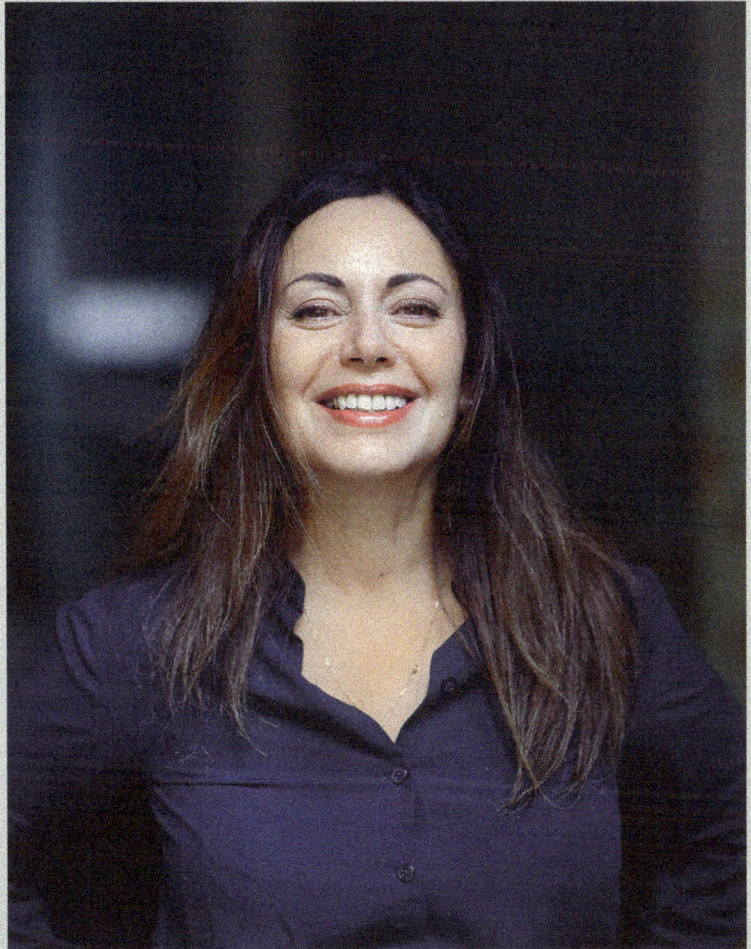

Arielle Artsztein learned to love food in France and today runs her own successful macaron bakery in Berlin.

lot. Even as she was truly enjoying eating healthily for the first time in her life, it didn't occur to her to pursue something with it professionally. Instead, she pursued a career in filmmaking, studying at the prestigious German Film and Television Academy in Berlin. It was there, while working on a documentary about the Jewish community in Berlin, that she suddenly realized that she didn't want to be working in film anymore. She found it exhausting to work with so many people. She wanted to find a way to work independently.

Then she discovered macarons. During a visit to Paris, she had one that was less than satisfactory, and she thought, "I could do better." So when she returned home to Berlin, she began experimenting in her kitchen. She quickly realized she had a knack for making the fine French confections. She began to devote every spare minute to making them. Her daughter was the first to notice that she seemed to enjoy baking macarons more than her actual job. She spent two years developing the perfect recipe and at the beginning of 2013 she opened her own store in the West Berlin neighborhood of Charlottenburg, which she simply called Arielle's Macarons. There you can enjoy classics like vanilla and dark chocolate as well as more exotic flavors like matcha and peach-lavender—all of them halal and kosher, and their preparation approved by Rabbi Schlomo Afanasev.

CHOLENT —BEEF STEW WITH BEANS AND BARLEY

SERVES 4
PREPARATION: 25 MIN.
SOAKING TIME: 12 HRS.
COOKING TIME: 2 ½ HRS.

BEEF STEW
¾ cup (150 g) dried white
  beans
1 lb (500 g) waxy potatoes
2 medium (200 g) carrots
2 large onions
3 cloves of garlic, peeled
  and crushed
3 tablespoons vegetable oil
1 ½ lb (600 g) of marbled
  beef for braising,
  chopped into large
  chunks
Salt
2 marrow bones
¾ cup (100 g) rolled barley
1 bay leaf
4 eggs
Freshly ground black
  pepper

BEEF STEW

1. Soak the beans overnight in a pot of cold water.

2. Preheat the oven to 325°F.

3. Prepare the vegetables first. Wash and peel the potatoes and cut them into bite-sized pieces. Place the potatoes in cold water. Peel the carrots, cut them in half or quarters lengthwise and cut them into pieces about 2-inches long. Peel the onions, halve them, and cut them into strips. Peel and crush the garlic cloves and set aside.

4. Heat the vegetable oil in a Dutch oven pot. Add the beef and cook until browned on all sides. Next, salt the pieces, remove from the pot and set aside. Add the onions and crushed garlic to the pot and cook for about 5 minutes until golden brown. Return the meat to the pot. Drain and add the potatoes and beans. Add the carrots, marrow bones, rolled barley, and bay leaf. Mix everything together.

5. Wash the eggs and place them in the pot. Then fill the pot with enough water to cover everything. Season well with salt and freshly ground pepper and bring a boil. Cover with a lid and put in the oven, allowing it to simmer for about 2 ½ hours until the meat and beans are tender. Then remove the eggs, peel, and season the stew with salt and freshly ground pepper to taste.

TO SERVE
Divide the beef stew among 4 bowls and serve each with 1 peeled egg

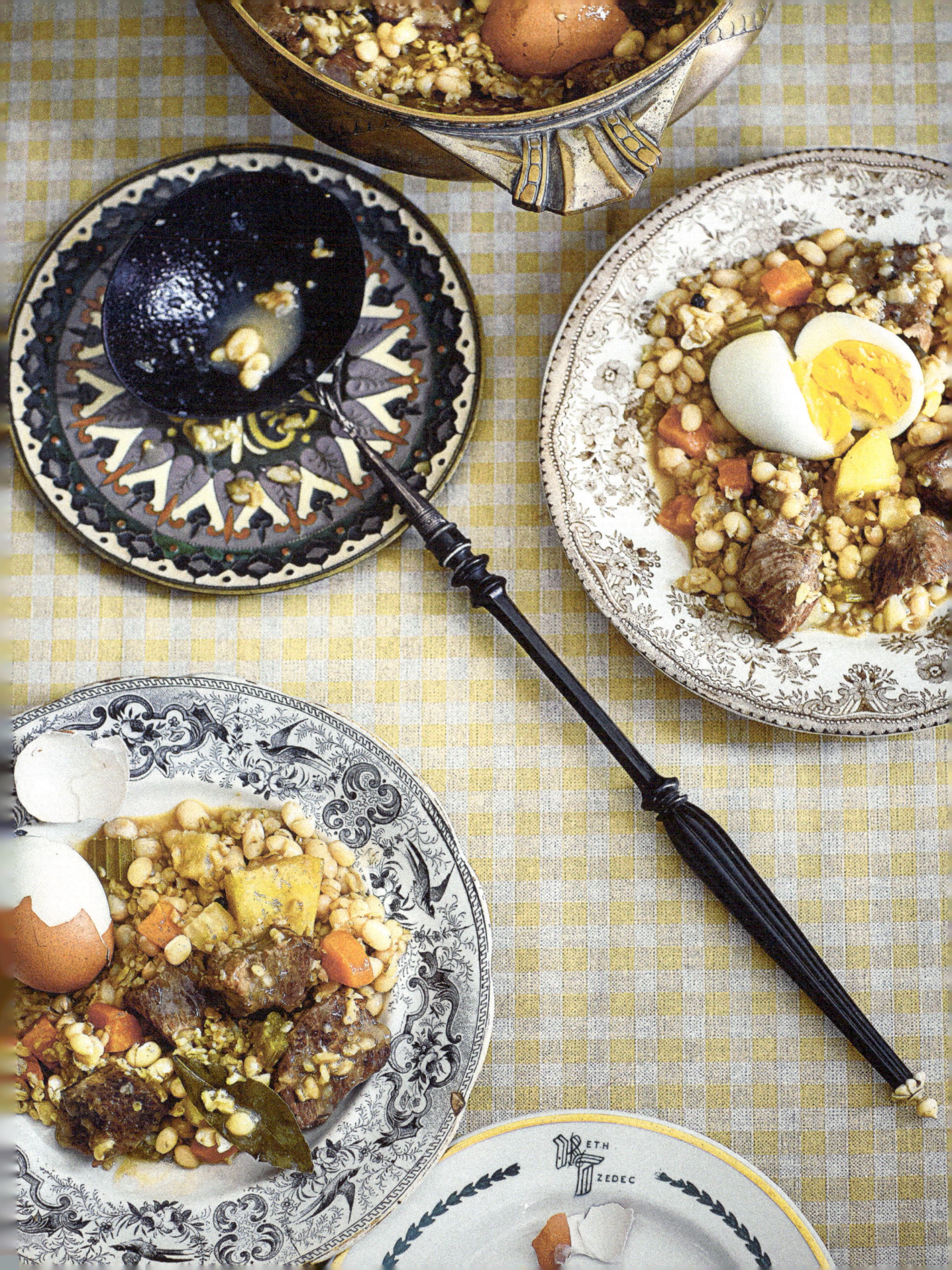

CARPE À LA JUIVE —CARP WITH STOCK AND HORSERADISH

SERVES 4
PREPARATION: 70 MIN.

CARP STOCK
4 fresh carp fillets
1 fresh carp head
1 small onion
1 stick of celery
½ leek (white part only)
½ bulb of fennel
1 small parsnip
1 medium carrot
1 bay leaf
½ teaspoon fennel seed
½ cup (1 ½ oz / 100 mL) Pernod
    (anise liqueur)
Salt
Freshly ground white pepper
Juice of 1 lemon

TO SERVE
4 teaspoons sour cream
1 piece of fresh horseradish root
    (3/4 inch), finely grated
Fresh parsley, to garnish
Baguette

This recipe is an homage to an old Jewish carp dish passed down from the Alsace region. Traditionally, the stock was boiled until all the collagen from the fish bones was cooked and the stock gelled as it cooled. This method, however, has a tendency to make the stock mustier in flavor. In this slightly quicker version, the carp is served lukewarm with a lighter stock. Unlike most carp dishes, this recipe is also suitable for the warmer months of the year.

CARP STOCK

1. Wash the carp fillets and the carp head and place in a large pot. Peel and halve the onion. Wash the celery, leek, and fennel bulb and cut into thirds. Peel the parsnip and carrot. Add the vegetables to the fish in the pot, along with the bay leaf, fennel seeds, and Pernod. Fill the pot with just enough lukewarm water to cover everything. Slowly bring the stock to a boil, skimming off any foam that rises to the surface. Allow to gently simmer for 10 minutes, then remove from the heat and let steep for another 30 minutes.
2. Carefully remove the carp fillets, carrot, and parsnip from the stock without breaking them up and place them on a plate. Cover with clear plastic wrap and set aside. Using a cheese cloth, carefully pour the stock into a pot. Season with salt, freshly ground white pepper and a little lemon juice and let it cool. Slice the cooked carrot and the parsnip.

TO SERVE

Place 1 carp fillet each on 4 shallow bowls and arrange with carrots and parsnip slices. Place 1 dollop of sour cream on each and sprinkle with freshly grated horseradish. Pour a little of the carp stock and garnish with parsley. Serve with a baguette slice, if desired.

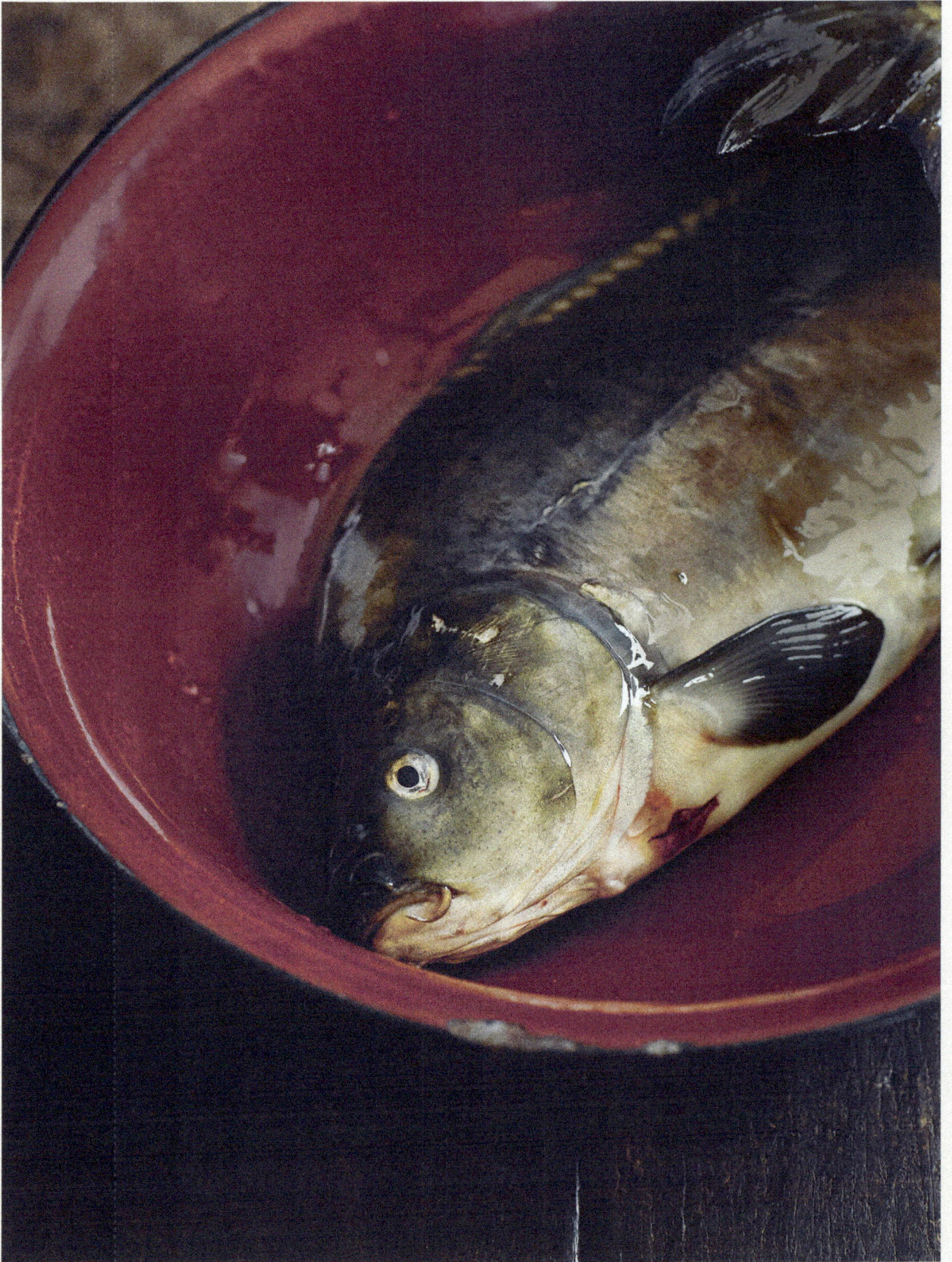

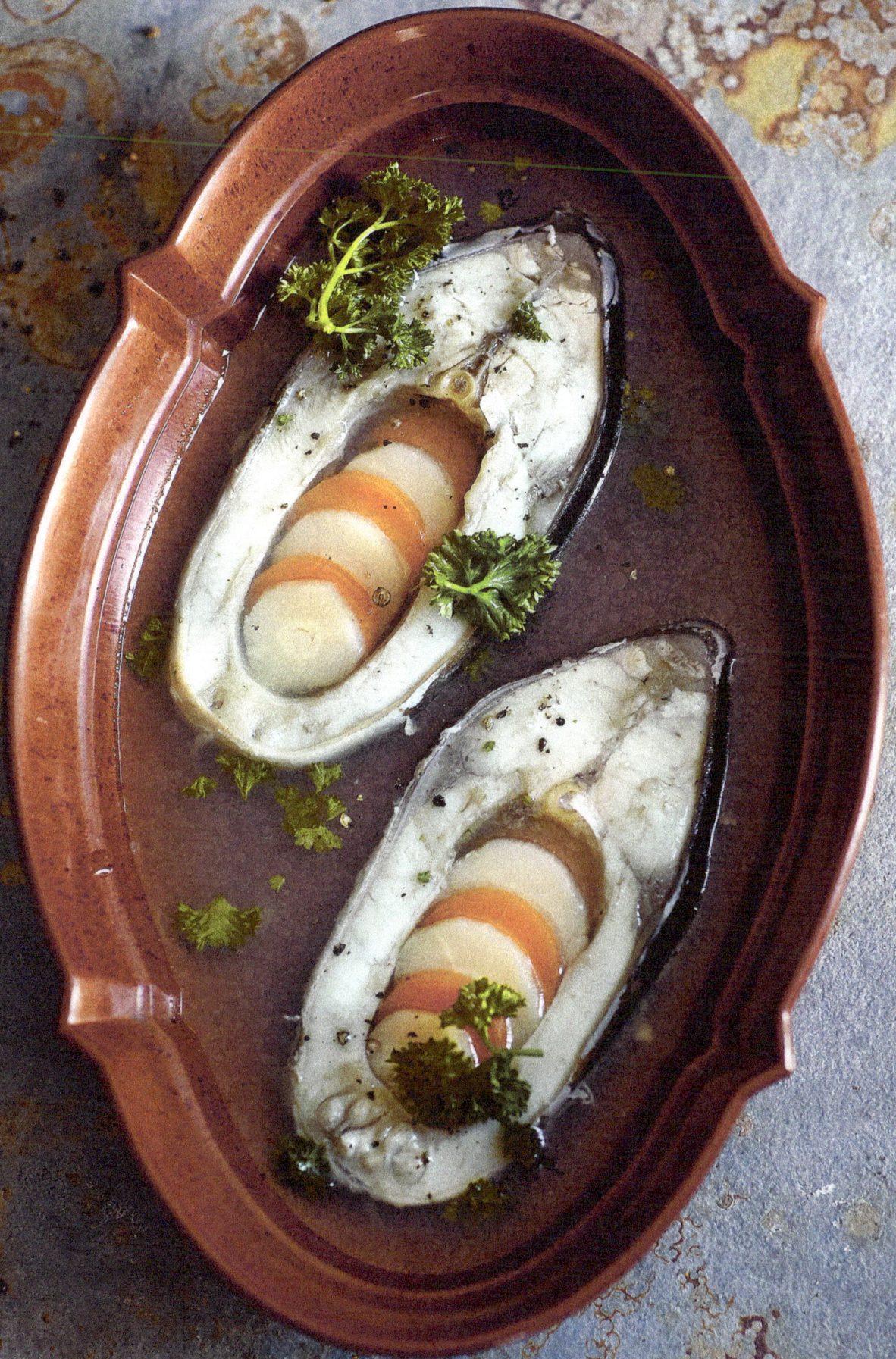

CHOPPED LIVER WITH EGGS

SERVES 4
PREPARATION: 20 MIN.

LIVER
2 eggs
2 medium (250 g) onions
2 tablespoons vegetable
  oil
9 oz (250 g) chicken liver
Salt
Freshly ground black
  pepper
A little wine vinegar

TO SERVE
4 slices of dark rye bread
  (see "Rye Loaf" on p. 46)
Butter
Chives, chopped
Pickled gherkins

LIVER

1. Hard boil the eggs for 9 minutes, rinse with cold water, peel and finely chop.
2. Meanwhile, cut the onions into thin strips. Heat the vegetable oil over medium-high heat in a pan and sweat the onions until translucent. Rinse the chicken livers thoroughly under running water and pat dry. Cut into large pieces and add to the pan with the onions. Increase the temperature slightly and cook for 5 minutes until the liver is cooked through and the onions are golden brown, season generously with salt and freshly ground pepper.
3. Transfer the liver and onion mixture to a cutting board. Chop everything with a knife until a creamy spread is formed. Mix in half of the chopped eggs and season again with salt, pepper, and a dash of vinegar.

TO SERVE

Spread the bread slices first with butter, then with the chopped liver. Spread the remaining chopped eggs on top and sprinkle with the chopped chives. Serve with pickled gherkins.

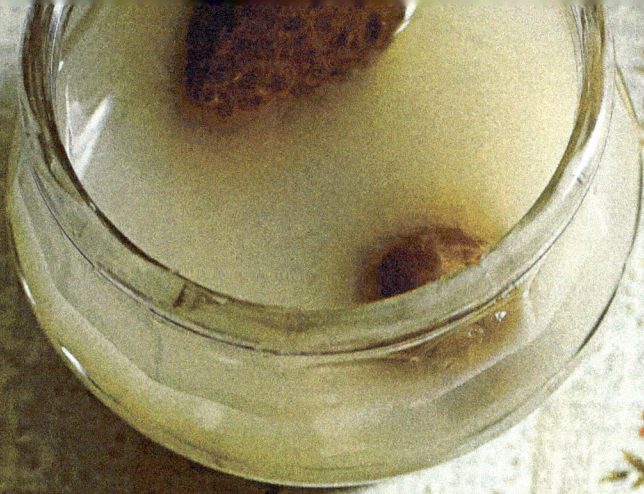

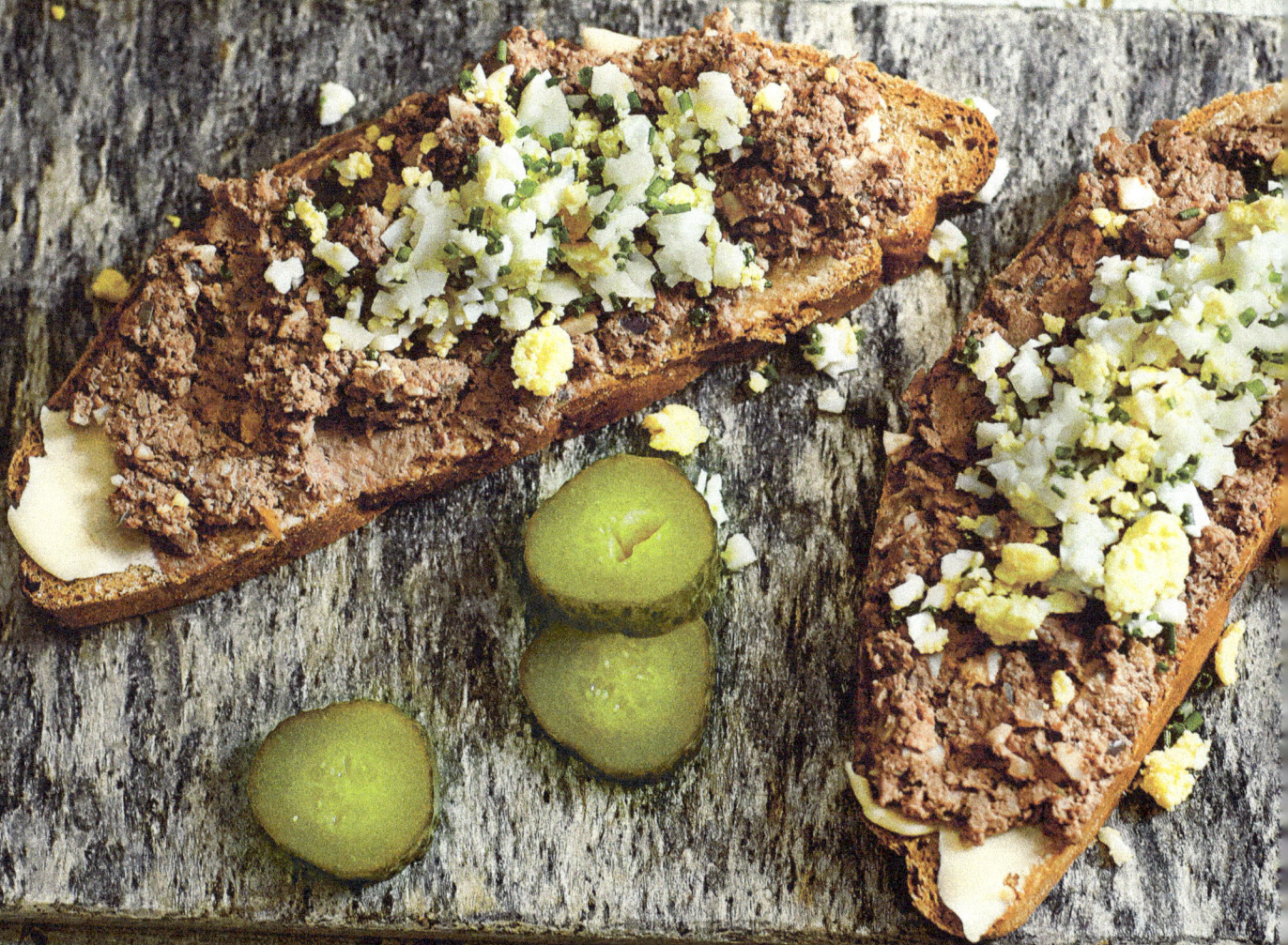

GRIBENES
—CRISPY CHICKEN SKIN
WITH BOILED POTATOES

SERVES 4
PREPARATION: 35 MIN.

GRIBENES

5 ½ oz (150 g) chicken skin
3 ½ oz (100 g) chicken or
 duck fat
1 lb (500 g) waxy potatoes
Salt
Handful (10 g) fresh
 marjoram, coarsely
 chopped
Freshly ground black
 pepper
Butter
Chives, chopped
Pickled gherkins

GRIBENES

1. Peel the potatoes, cut in half or quarters depending on size, and cook in salted water for 20-25 minutes.

2. While the potatoes are cooking, prepare the chicken. Start by washing the chicken skin, pat dry, and cut into thin strips. Heat the chicken or duck fat in a skillet. Add the chicken skin and cook over medium-high heat until the skin is nicely crisped, about 10 minutes. Allow the chicken skin to cool slightly in the fat.

3. Once the potatoes are done cooking, drain the water and mix with the chicken skin and some of the fat. Then sprinkle with coarsely chopped marjoram, salt and pepper.

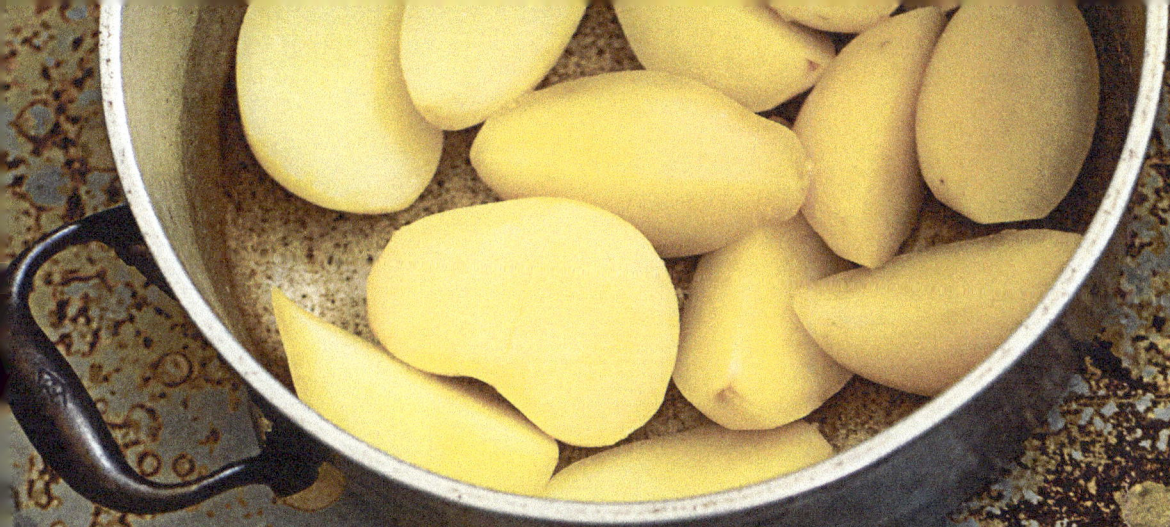

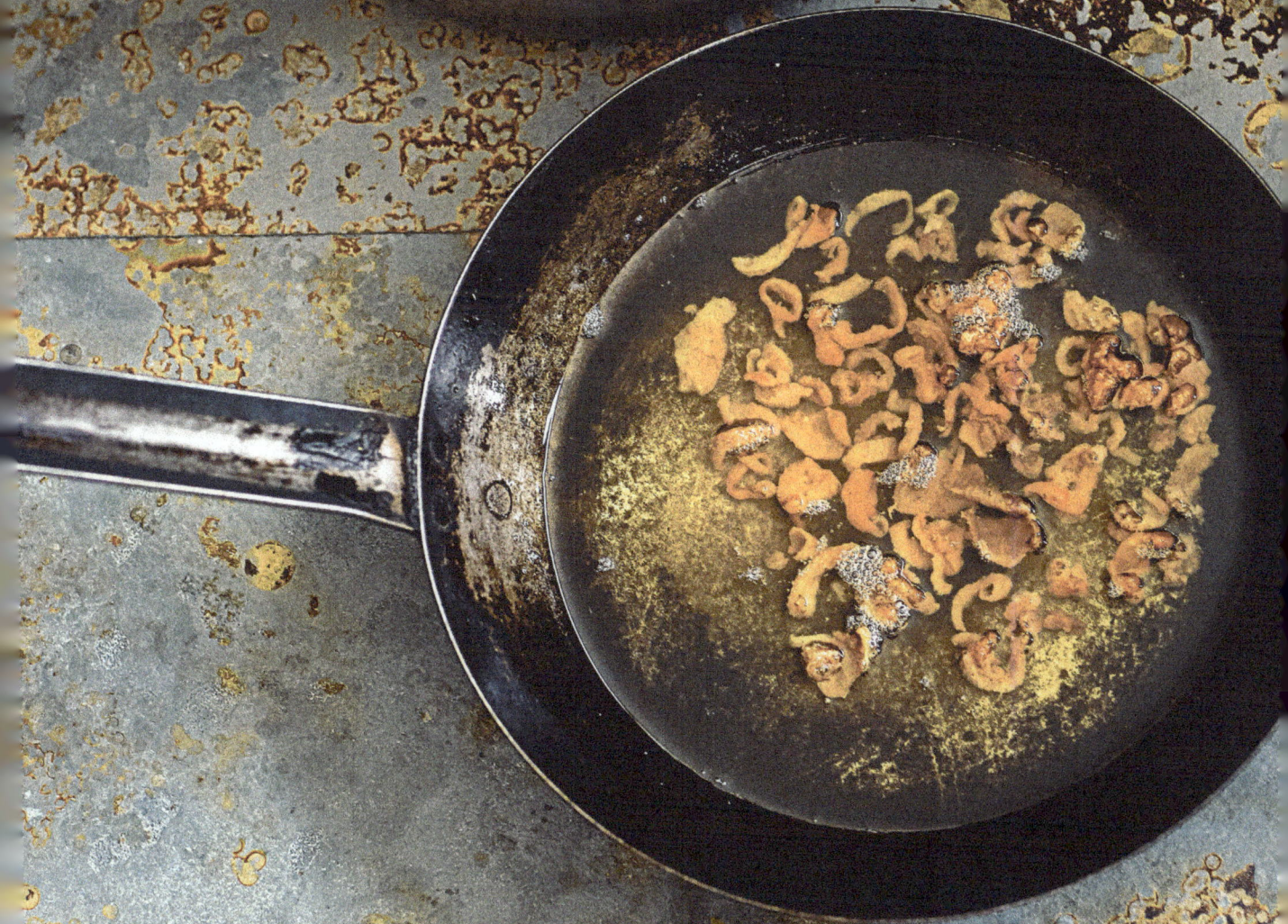

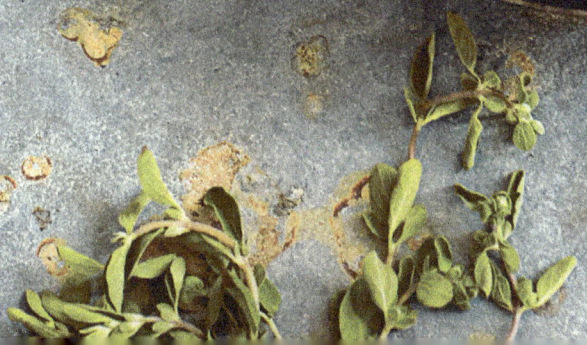

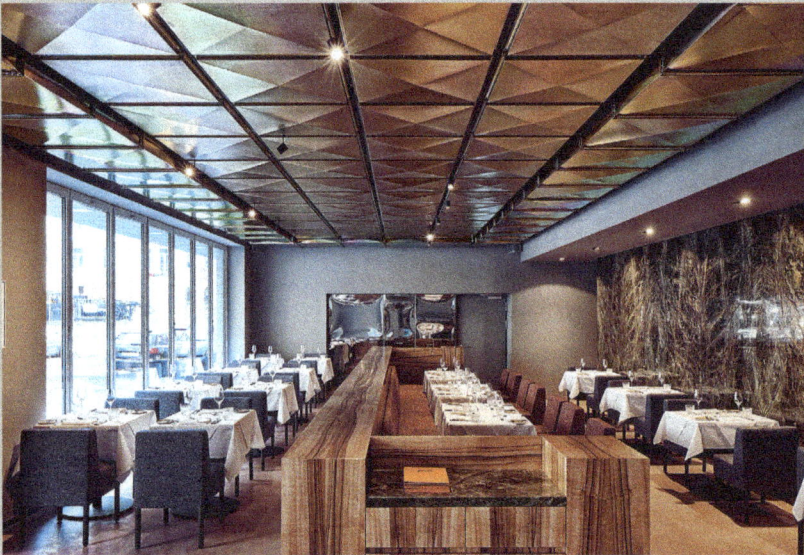

responsible for several gastronomical ventures: the Stanley and Shuka bars and café, and an event and catering company.

James and David have never consciously billed themselves as "Jewish" restaurateurs. It's not as if they were trying to hide it. At the same time, they were conscious of their grandparent's relationship to the German past and that meant a different understanding of what it meant to be Jewish and German. As they put it, "We grew up as Jews in Germany, our grandparents survived the Holocaust." In their family that meant that their grandparents drew strict boundaries with non-Jewish Germans. "We live here, but we're not German," James and David explain. Intoning the words of their family, they add, "German friends are okay, but definitely not a German girlfriend or German wife." Only

later did James and David come to view themselves as something less apart from their non-Jewish, German friends and neighbors. James and David were not "Jews in Germany"; they were German Jews. Still, it's a complicated negotiation. It was for those reasons that it wasn't until recently that the brothers were more open about their Jewish heritage. That changed, though, after the opening of Maxie Eisen, when the Frankfurter Allgemeine Zeitung wrote a full-page story about it in which they stressed the brother's status as Jewish. A lot of Germans reacted positively to the piece. But others responded with anti-Semitic comments. That's when they decided, "We'll make no secret of it now" and consciously sought to be up front about it and work with it. They also wanted to make a statement: Jewish cuisine can compete with other world cuisines, something the brothers have more than proven.

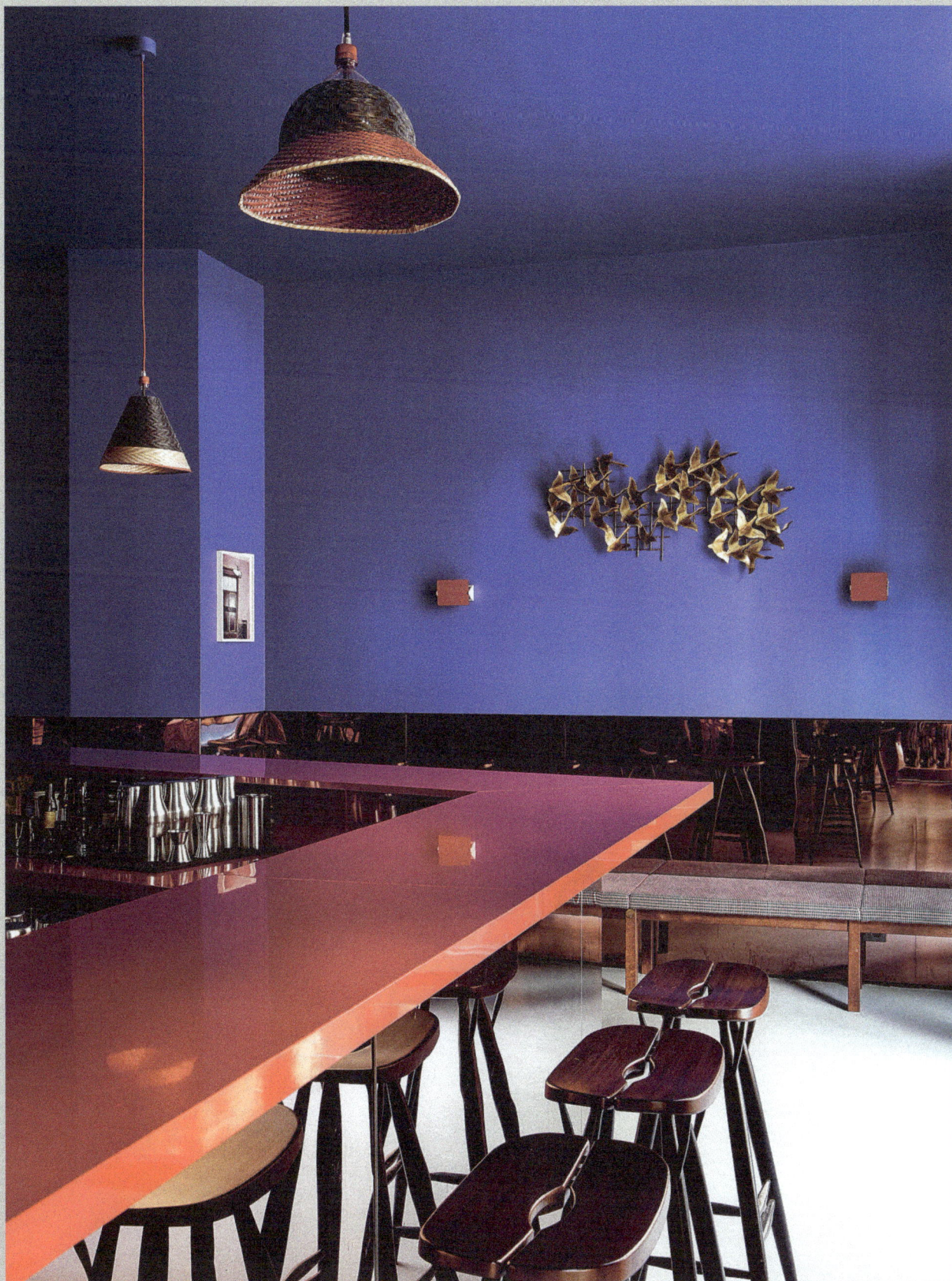

CHICKEN STOCK

FOR 1 1/3 quarts (1.2 L)
PREPARATION: 20 MIN.
COOKING TIME: 3 HRS.

CHICKEN STOCK
1 chicken (2-3 lb)
1 stalk of celery
1 medium carrot
1 leek
1 onion
1 clove garlic
Handful of fresh parsley
3 black peppercorns
1 sprig of thyme
1 bay leaf salt
Freshly ground black
  pepper

STOCK

1. Rinse the chicken under cold running water. Place in a large pot, cover completely with about 2 ½ quarts of cold water. Bring to a slow boil, skimming off the foam with a ladle or spoon.

2. In the meantime, prepare the vegetables. Peel the celery and the carrot and cut them into very large pieces. Clean the leek, wash and chop into large pieces. Remove only the outermost layer of skin from the onion and cut the onion in half crosswise. Crush the unpeeled garlic clove with the blade of a knife. Wash the parsley, finely chop, and set aside.

3. Add the vegetables, garlic, peppercorns, and herbs to the pot and simmer gently for another 2 ½ hours.

4. As soon as the bones of the chicken start to separate from the meat, the stock is ready. Line a fine-mesh strainer with a damp cheese cloth, add the parsley, and strain the stock through it. Return the chicken stock to a low boil and reduce to 1 1/3 quarts. When done, season with salt and freshly ground pepper.

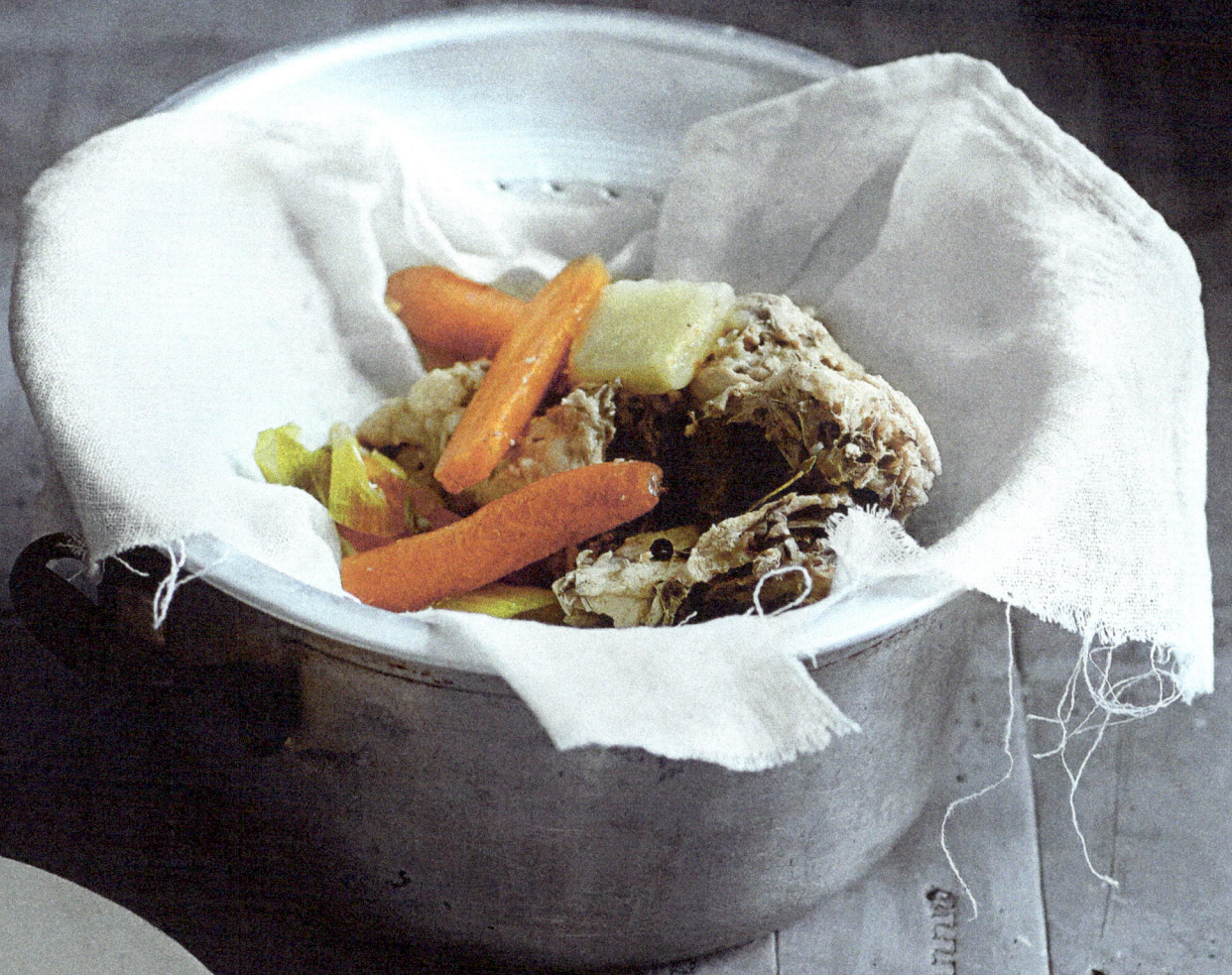

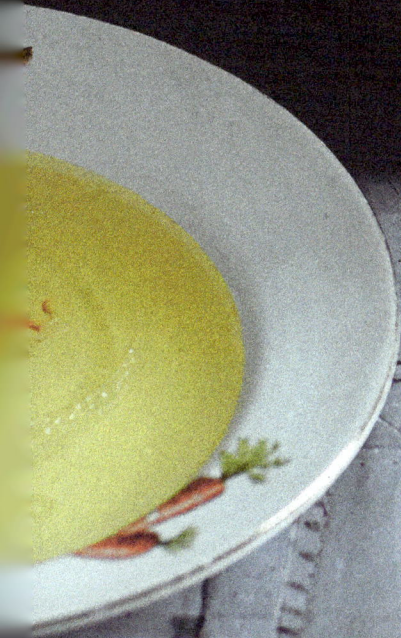

CHICKEN SOUP WITH MATZO BALLS

SERVES 4/ MAKES 20
    SMALL MATZO BALLS
PREPARATION: 30 MIN.
SOAKING TIME: 1 HR.

MATZO BALLS
1 small onion
4 tablespoons (55 g)
    butter
1-inch piece (10 g) fresh
    ginger
½ cup (20 g) flat-leaf
    parsley
1 organic lemon
2 cups (240 g) matzo meal
2 eggs, beaten
1 pinch of cayenne pepper
Salt
Freshly ground black
    pepper

CHICKEN SOUP
1 small carrot
1 small leek
1 1/3 quarts (1.2 L) chicken
    stock (see recipe on p.
    120)
Salt

MATZO BALLS

Peel and finely dice the onion. Melt the butter in a small pot and sweat the chopped onions in it until translucent. Allow the onions to cool. Peel the ginger and grate it into a large bowl. Wash the parsley, pat dry, finely chop the leaves and add to the bowl. Wash the lemon in hot water, zest or grate ¼ of the peel and add it to the bowl. Add the matzo meal, cooked onions, whisked eggs, cayenne pepper, and a generous pinch of salt and freshly ground pepper. Mix everything together, cover and place in the refrigerator for 1 hour.

CHICKEN SOUP

1. In the meantime, peel the carrot and clean and wash the leek. Julienne the vegetables into matchstick pieces. Set aside.
2. Bring the chicken stock to a boil. Remove the matzo dough from the refrigerator. With moistened hands, form 20 small balls. Slide into the hot stock and gently simmer for 10-15 minutes. Five minutes before it is finished simmering, add the vegetables. Season with salt to taste.

TO SERVE

Divide the soup among 4 bowls and serve hot.

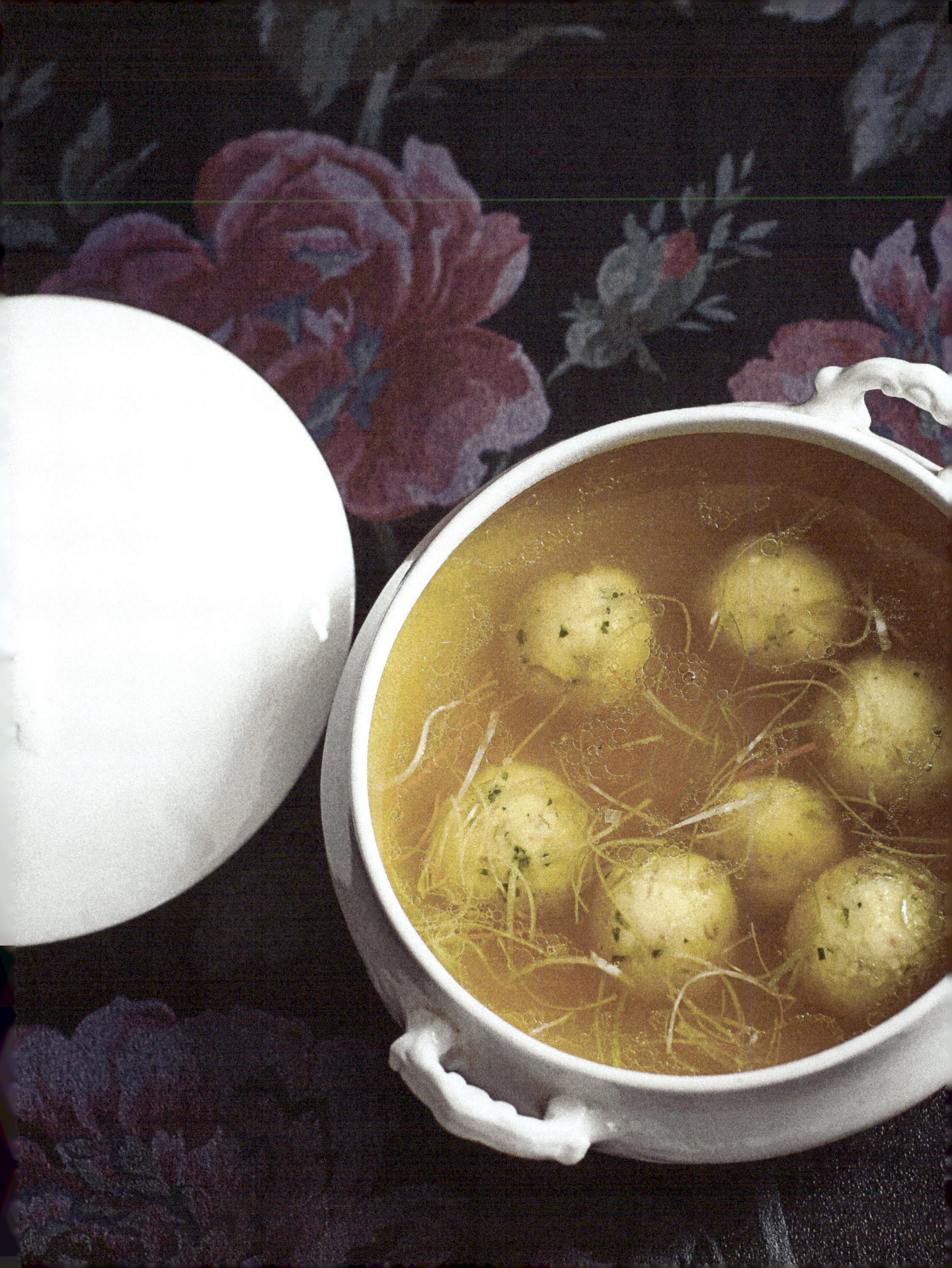

KNISHES WITH POTATO & GOUDA FILLING

MAKES ABOUT 24 KNISHES
PREPARATION: 60 MIN.
RESTING TIME: 60 MIN.
BAKING TIME: 20-25 MIN.

DOUGH
2 cups (250 g) pastry flour
1 teaspoon baking powder
1 pinch of salt
2 tablespoons, plus 1 teaspoon vegetable
    oil
2 eggs

FILLING
1 lb (400 g) potatoes
Salt
1 red onion
1 tablespoon neutral vegetable oil
½ teaspoon cumin seeds
2/3 cup (80 g) Gouda, grated
Freshly ground black pepper

FINAL STEPS
Pastry flour for work surface
1 egg
1 egg yolk
2 tablespoons milk
Sesame seeds, black cumin seeds, and
    coarse sea salt

DOUGH

Mix the flour, baking powder, and 1 pinch of salt in a bowl and place on a large wooden board or work surface. Form a well in the center, add the eggs and vegetable oil and knead everything vigorously for 10 minutes until the dough is elastic and slightly silky. Place the dough in a lightly oiled bowl, cover and let rest at room temperature for about 1 hour.

FILLING

In the meantime, wash, peel and halve the potatoes and boil in salted water for about 20 minutes until soft. Drain the water. Cut the onion into thin strips and sweat them in a pan with the vegetable oil for about 5 minutes until translucent. Roughly mash the potatoes with a fork, stir in the onions, cumin, and grated Gouda and season with salt and freshly ground pepper.

FINISH & BAKE

1. Preheat the oven to 350°F. Line a baking sheet with parchment paper.
2. Place the dough on a lightly floured work surface and roll out to a sheet about ½-inch thick. Cut out circles with 4 ½ inch diameters. Spoon 1 tablespoon of potato filling in the center of each. Lightly beat the egg and brush the edges of the dough with it. Fold the dough circles over the filling to form half-moons. Press the edges together with a fork and secure.
3. Place the filled pastries on the baking sheet. In a small bowl, mix the egg yolk with the milk until smooth and brush the knishes with it. Sprinkle with sesame seeds, black cumin seeds, and coarse sea salt to taste.
4. Bake the knishes for 20-25 minutes until golden brown and serve warm.

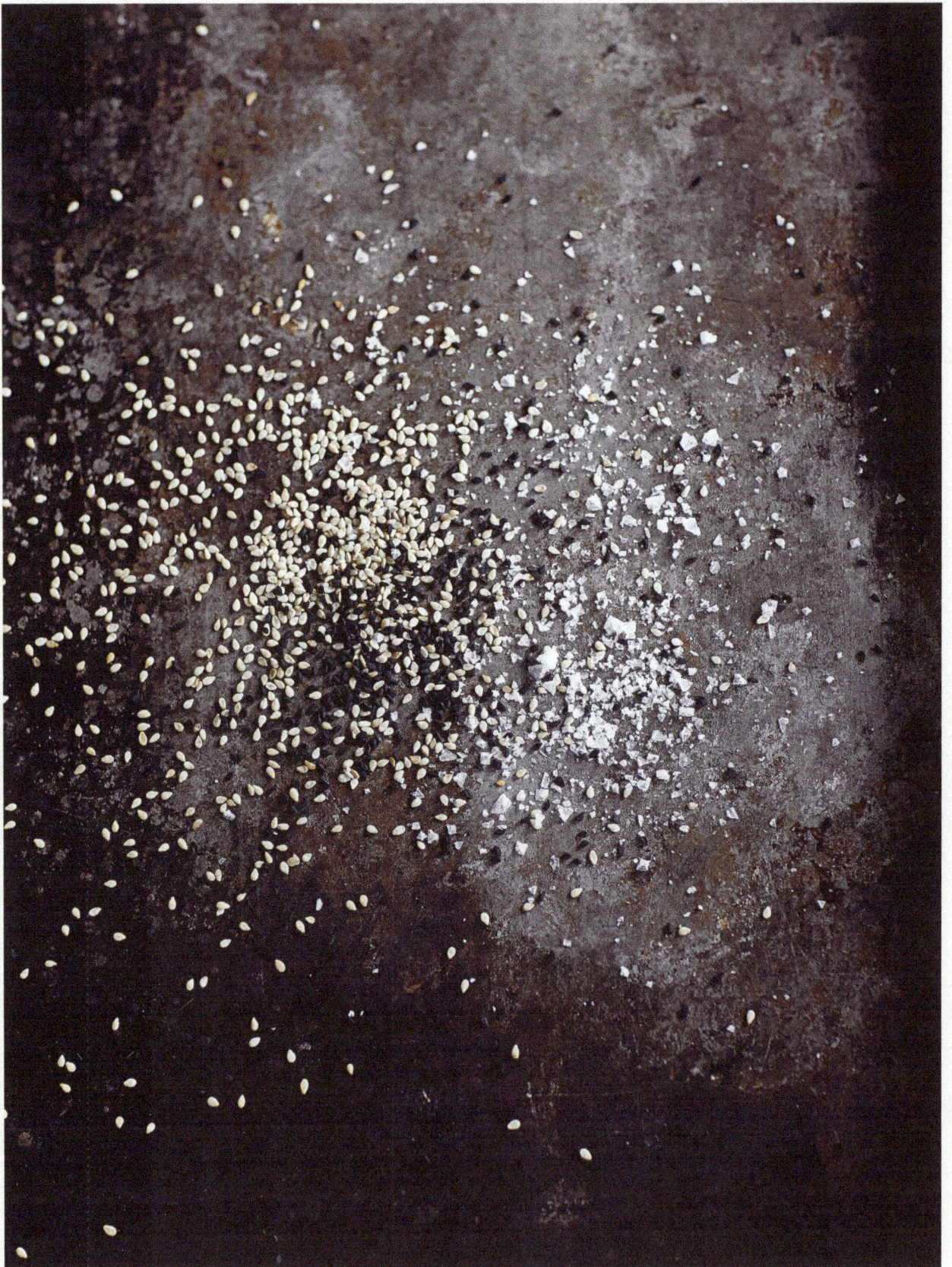

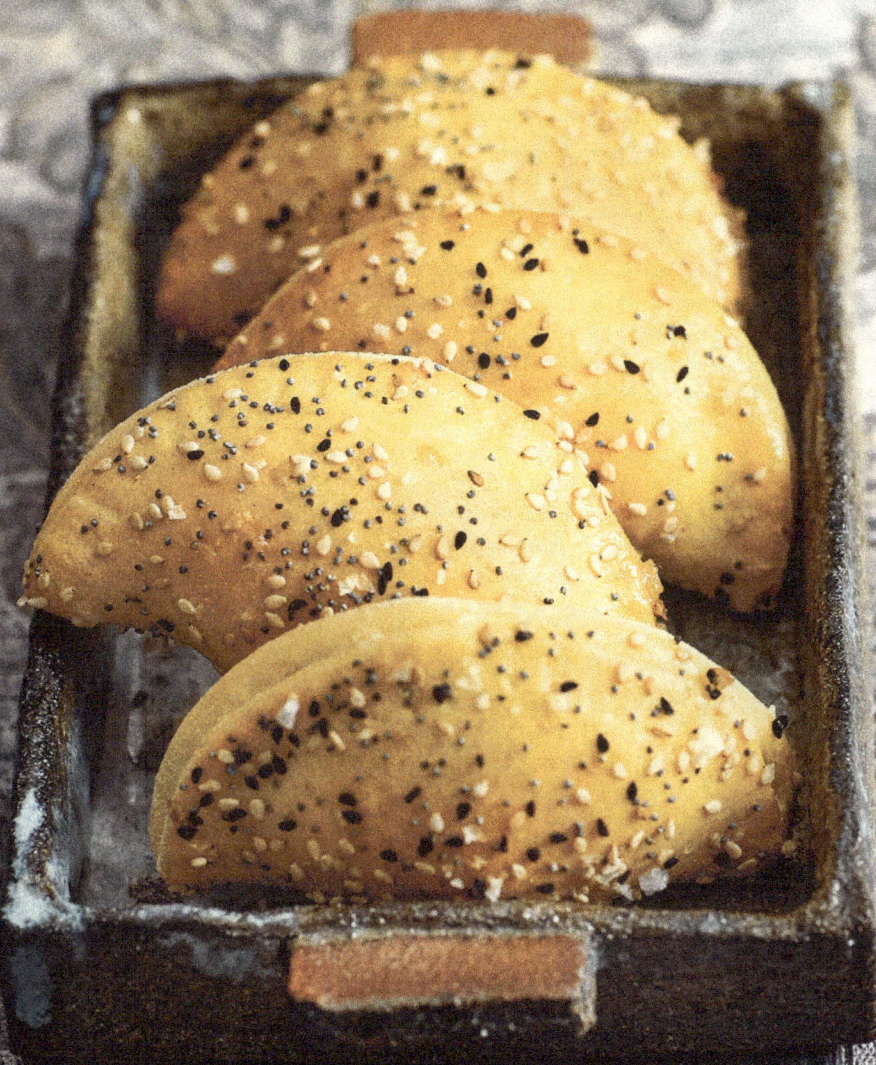

HAYA MOLCHO, Vienna

WORLD CUISINE IN THE FAMILY

Haya's likes to combine a lot of elements in her cooking, an extension of her upbringing in two countries and extensive travels. Haya was born in Tel Aviv but moved with her parents to Bremen, Germany when she was still a kid. Today she divides her time between Germany and Austria, where she runs her own chain of restaurants, known as Neni. Haya has a fun-loving and sincere demeanor, and she loves to talk about her family. She comes from a big family, and as with a lot of big Jewish families, cooking was a big part of her childhood. She describes how back then women were still largely responsible for most of the cooking. Usually, they did it together. Grandmas, aunts, nieces, and granddaughters threw themselves into the lively chaos of preparing food. These early influences may have shaped her relationship to food, but she has always found a way to reinvent even the most familiar of dishes from home. "Everyone interprets their mother's or grandmother's recipes in a new and different way," she observes, "You just use what's on hand. When I'm in Austria, for example, I cook with 'beetle beans' because they're available here. But I'll serve them with tahini and seed oil." A mixture of Occident and Orient.

After Haya moved to Bremen, her family continued to cook Israeli food, but there were far fewer fresh vegetables in Germany than they had enjoyed in Israel. Whenever anyone from Israel would visit, they would ask them to bring fresh vegetables: "We didn't ask for flowers or toys, but tomatoes, watermelons, and cucumbers. Our longing for home was strong."

Even as she is still attached to the foods from home, she's always been curious about other cuisines. Not long after she married, she and her husband, Sammy, traveled the world, living like nomads for seven years. That's how she got to know and love so many different

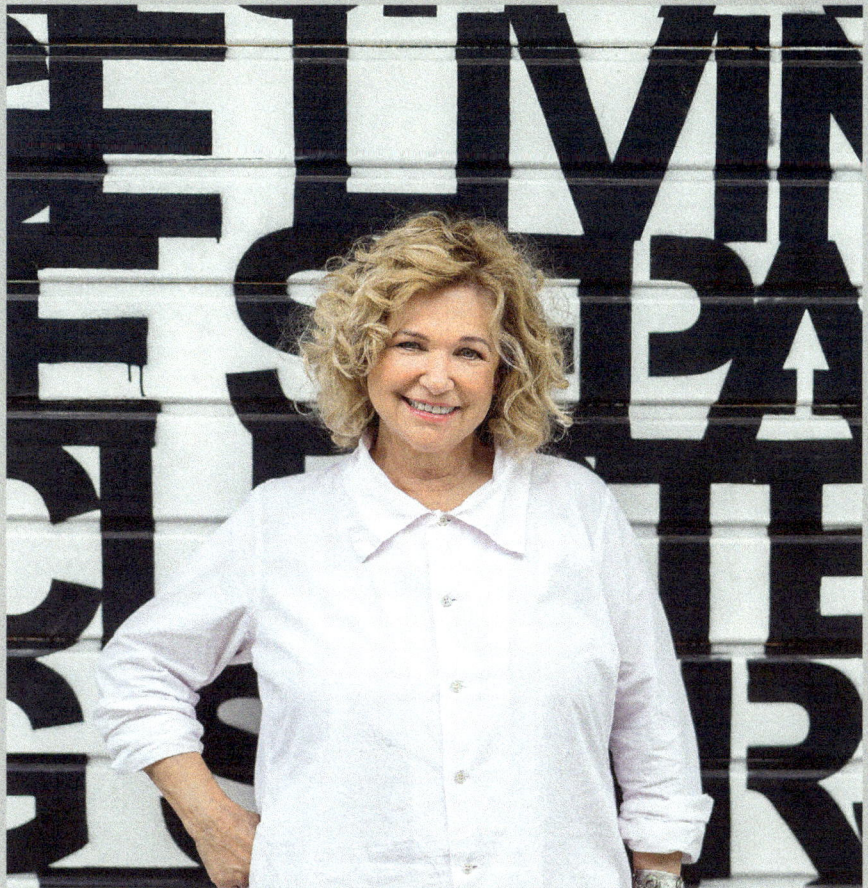

Food means family to Haya Molcho. She runs her restaurant business with her sons.

types of cuisines, from Japanese to Moroccan to Indian. No matter where they were, Haya was always cooking, checking out the markets, talking to traders, and gathering all the knowledge she could. Through those years of intensive exploration, she developed an abiding respect and appreciation for the world's diverse food cultures.

Another major source of influence on her cooking, is her family's Romanian origins. Jews from Romania, she says, are very fond of pickling vegetables. Even now, whenever cucumbers, tomatoes, or herbs are in season Haya is sure to make time to devote to pickling. Haya also continues to cook meatballs in a tomato sauce, in the Romanian way that her mother used to prepare them. She adds her own touch, though, integrating different flavors like the North African spice blend, ras el hanout. At her restaurant, Neni, she has also featured Romanian specialties like zacusca,

which is a bit like baba ghanoush only it's made with peppers instead of eggplant.

There is no such thing as Jewish or Israeli cuisine, Haya maintains. They are both world cuisines. "People moved to Israel and brought their culinary cultures with them. That means recipes from Yemen, India, Ethiopia, Russia, or Poland! It's all Jewish food! These different influences all make Israeli cuisine, a world cuisine."

Even so, there are certain ingredients and dishes that characterize the culinary culture in Israel. Preserved lemons, for instance, are the backbone of Israeli cuisine, and she makes them herself. Nice and sour, a bit sweet and very salty, they are extremely easy to prepare and keep for a very long time. They taste good chopped up in fresh salads or in a sandwich or added whole into soups. In Israel, you simply can't imagine life without

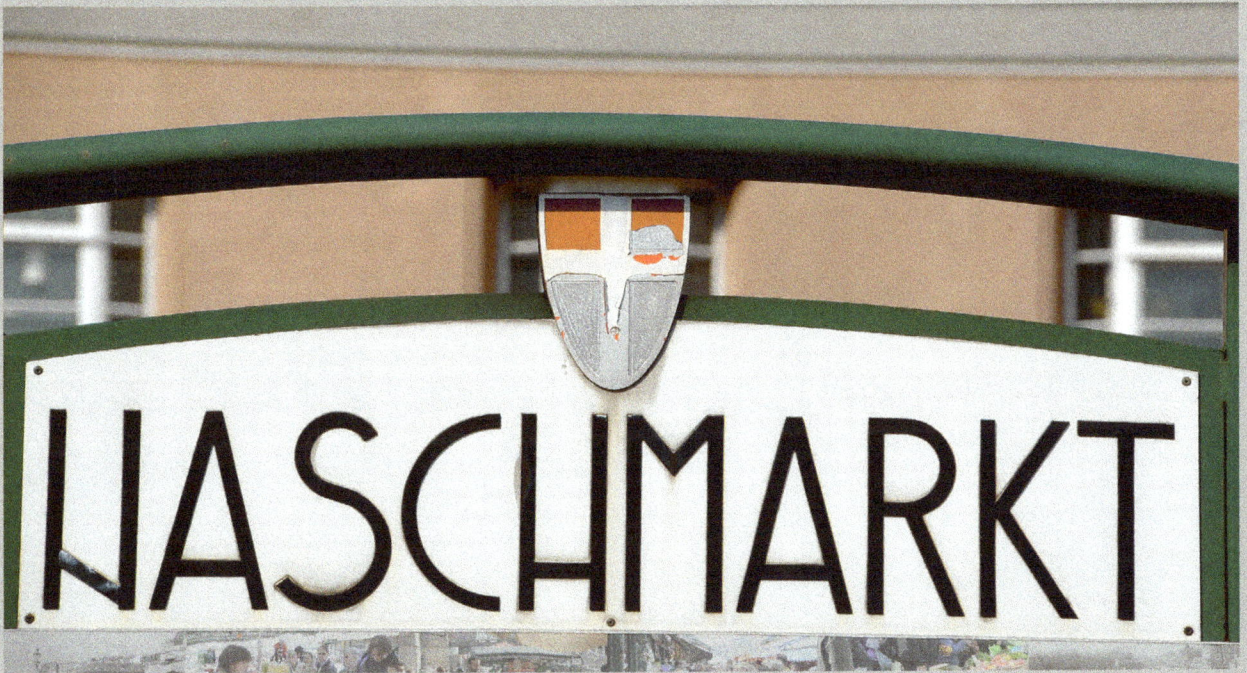

Top: Neni is located at the Naschmarkt in Vienna.
Right side: Also at the Naschmarkt, the majolica house by Otto Wagner.

them. An equally iconic dish is baba ghanoush: a dip made from smoked eggplant. Baba ghanoush can be found in many cuisines, from India to North Africa and, of course, throughout the Middle East. It combines many cultures, much like Haya herself. Incredibly aromatic, baba ghanoush is a popular dish at Neni and her personal favorite at home. It's the smoky aroma that sets it apart. The eggplants are cooked in a hot oven until their skin turns almost black. Although you remove the skin before preparing the dish, it leaves a lingering smoky note. The influence of Palestine on Israel cooking is another unifying element. "You can't," Haya notes, "underestimate the influence of Palestine. Israel has very much adapted Palestinian cuisine. Falafel, hummus, and so on. Israel then transformed them a bit, but the general inspiration comes from the Middle East."

Haya's cooking continues to draw on her Israeli upbringing. Some dishes remain as they are because

they were perfect even back then. But others she reinterprets. She likes, for instance, to play with tahini and falafel, creating rather unconventional dishes with them. At Neni they serve falafel in the classic, Middle Eastern way, but also in more experimental varieties like popcorn falafel, tuna falafel or lentil falafel. Haya's thinks that part of the fun of cooking is that everything can be reinvented, even as the Middle Eastern accent remains.

For Haya, traditional Jewish food is strongly tied to tradition and the holidays: "Longing, tradition, holidays, being at home—that's Jewish cuisine for me." Outside of the holidays, however, in her daily life, her cooking is most heavily influenced by her Israeli upbringing and her appreciation for it as a world cuisine. "Thank God!" she declares, "Because if you had a beautiful childhood, no one can take that away from you."

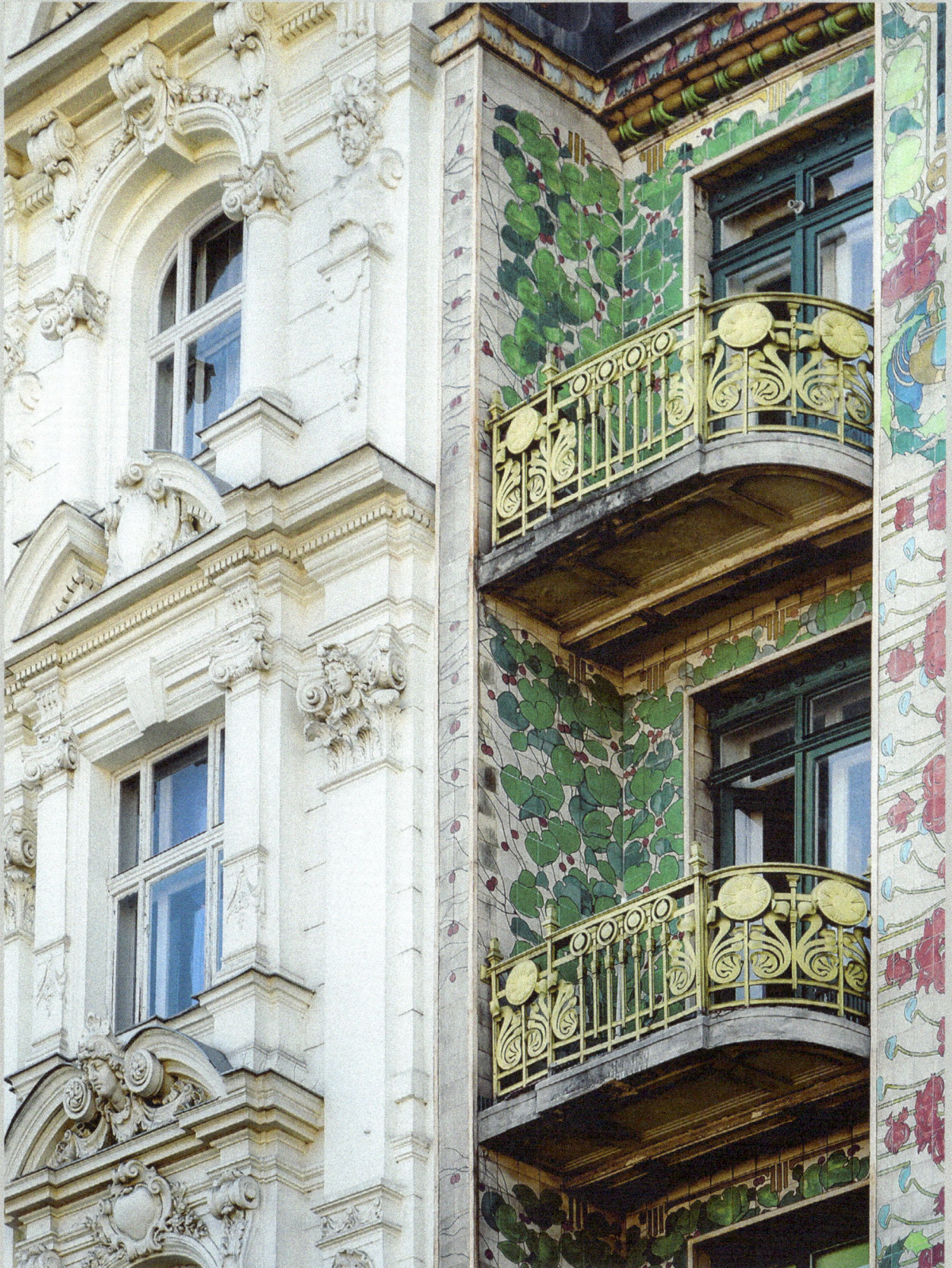

BABA GHANOUSH

SERVES 4
PREPARATION: 50 MIN.

EGGPLANT PURÉE
4 eggplants
4 cloves of garlic
1 cup (125 g) tahini
2 tablespoons olive oil
2 tablespoons lemon juice
Salt

TO SERVE
A little olive oil to drizzle
Black cumin seeds or
    za'atar (African spice
    mix)

EGGPLANT PURÉE

1. Heat the oven to its highest setting (400-450°F).
2. Wash the eggplants, place them on a baking sheet and roast for about 30-40 minutes until blackened and flesh is very soft. Turn the eggplants every 10 minutes so that all sides are evenly roasted.
3. Remove the tray from the oven and allow the eggplants to cool briefly. Then, while still hot, cut open lengthwise and use a spoon to loosen the soft flesh from the charred skin. Roughly chop the soft eggplant flesh and place in a bowl. Discard the stem ends and skins.
4. Finely grate the garlic cloves and add to the eggplant. Using a fork, mash the eggplant up a bit, then add the tahini, olive oil, and freshly squeezed lemon juice and mix until everything is well combined. Season with salt to taste.

TO SERVE

Scoop the baba ghanoush into a serving bowl and drizzle with olive oil. Garnish with optional black cumin seeds or za'atar.

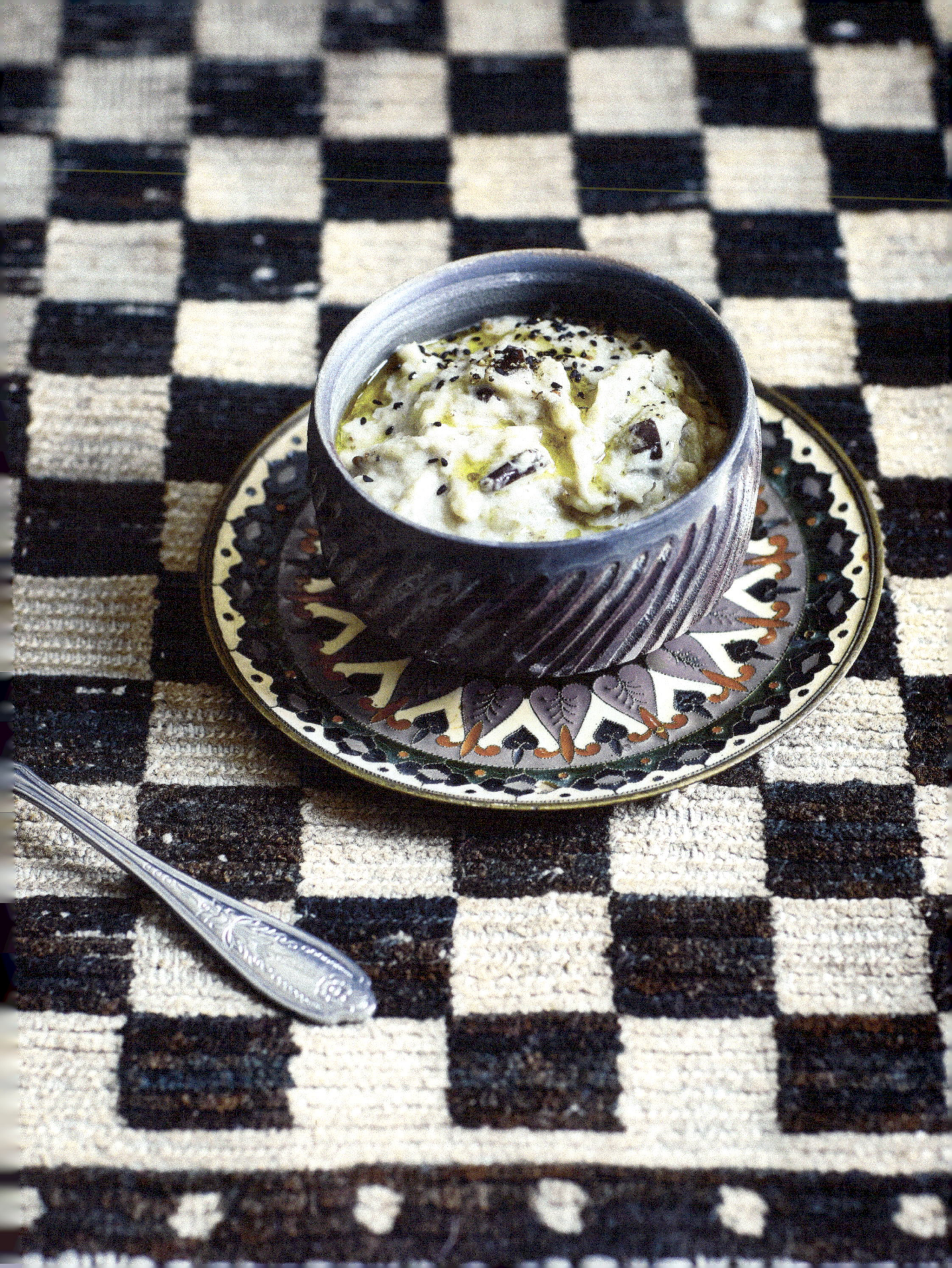

PRESERVED LEMONS

MAKES 1 LARGE JAR
PREPARATION: 10-15 MIN.
INFUSION TIME: 20 DAYS

PRESERVED LEMONS
6 organic lemons
1/3 cup (100 g) sea salt
1/3 cup (50 g) sugar
2 ¾ tablespoons (40 mL)
  olive oil

PRESERVED LEMONS

1. Squeeze the juice from 1 lemon into a bowl. Wash the remaining 5 lemons in hot water, rub dry, and cut into slices. Remove the seeds.

2. Mix the lemon slices with the sea salt, sugar, and lemon juice and leave to infuse for about 10 hours. Stir and mix the lemon slices every now and then.

3. When done infusing, stir once more, then pour everything into a jar and add in the olive oil. Close the jar tightly and leave the lemons to infuse in the refrigerator for 20 days. Shake the jar from time to time.

Tip: Preserved lemons taste great in stews like lamb or beef.

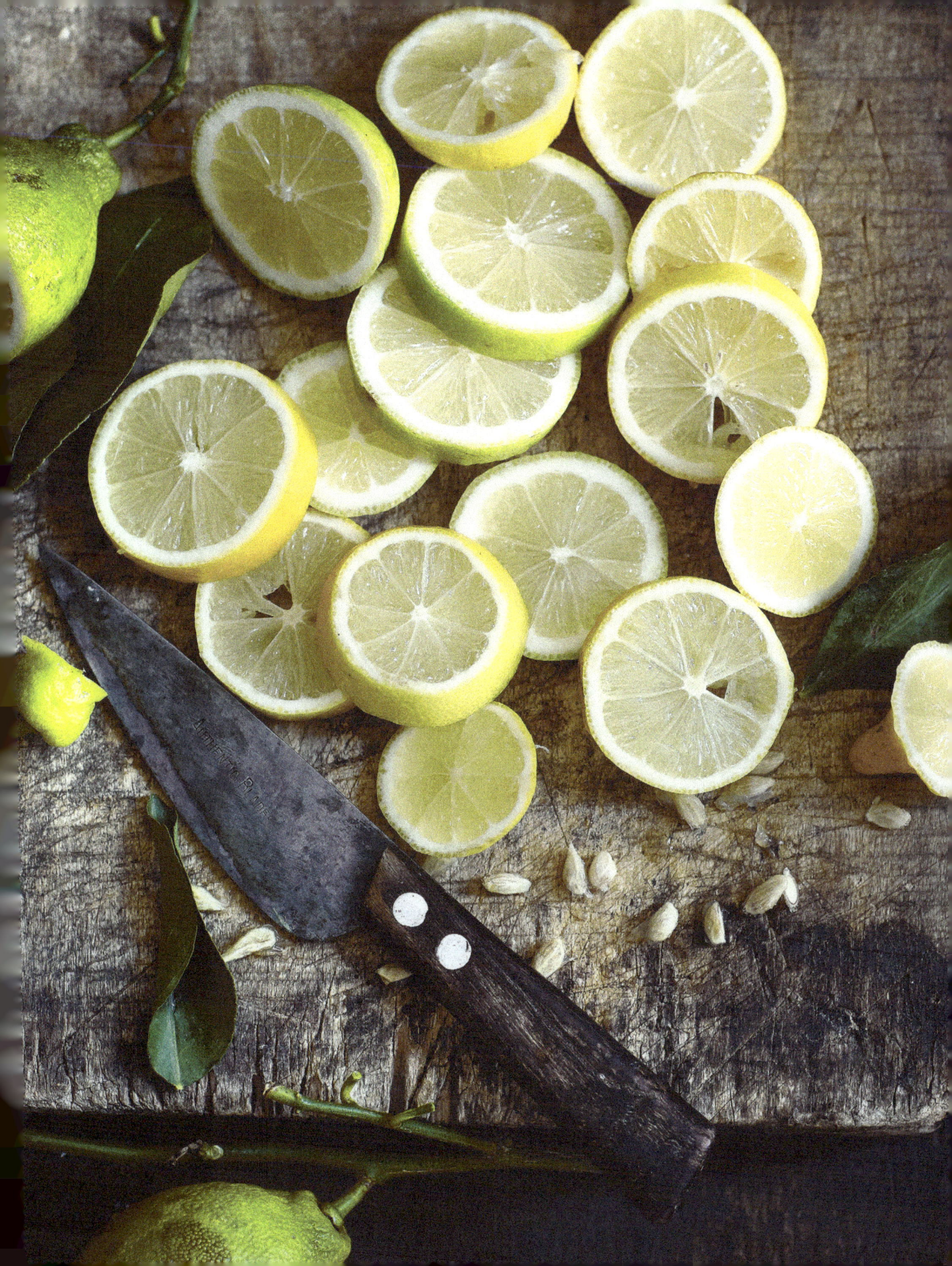

PICKLED CUCUMBERS

MAKES 2 LARGE JARS
PREPARATION: 10 MIN.
PICKLING TIME: 4 - 6
    DAYS

PICKLED CUCUMBERS
2 lb (1 kg) cucumbers
1 bunch of dill
2 chili peppers
4 cloves of garlic
3 tablespoons salt
1 teaspoon black
    peppercorns

PICKLED CUCUMBERS

1. Wash the cucumbers and cut them into finger-thick slices, including the peel. Divide the cucumber slices into 2 large canning jars.

2. Wash and roughly chop the dill sprigs. Divide the dill, chilies, and garlic cloves among the jars as well. Then add the salt and peppercorns and fill each jar with lukewarm water so that everything is well covered. Close the jars tightly and shake them a bit so that the contents mix well and leave them in a cold place for 4-6 days.

Tip: These pickled cucumbers go well with cured meat, chopped liver or even as an addition to salads.

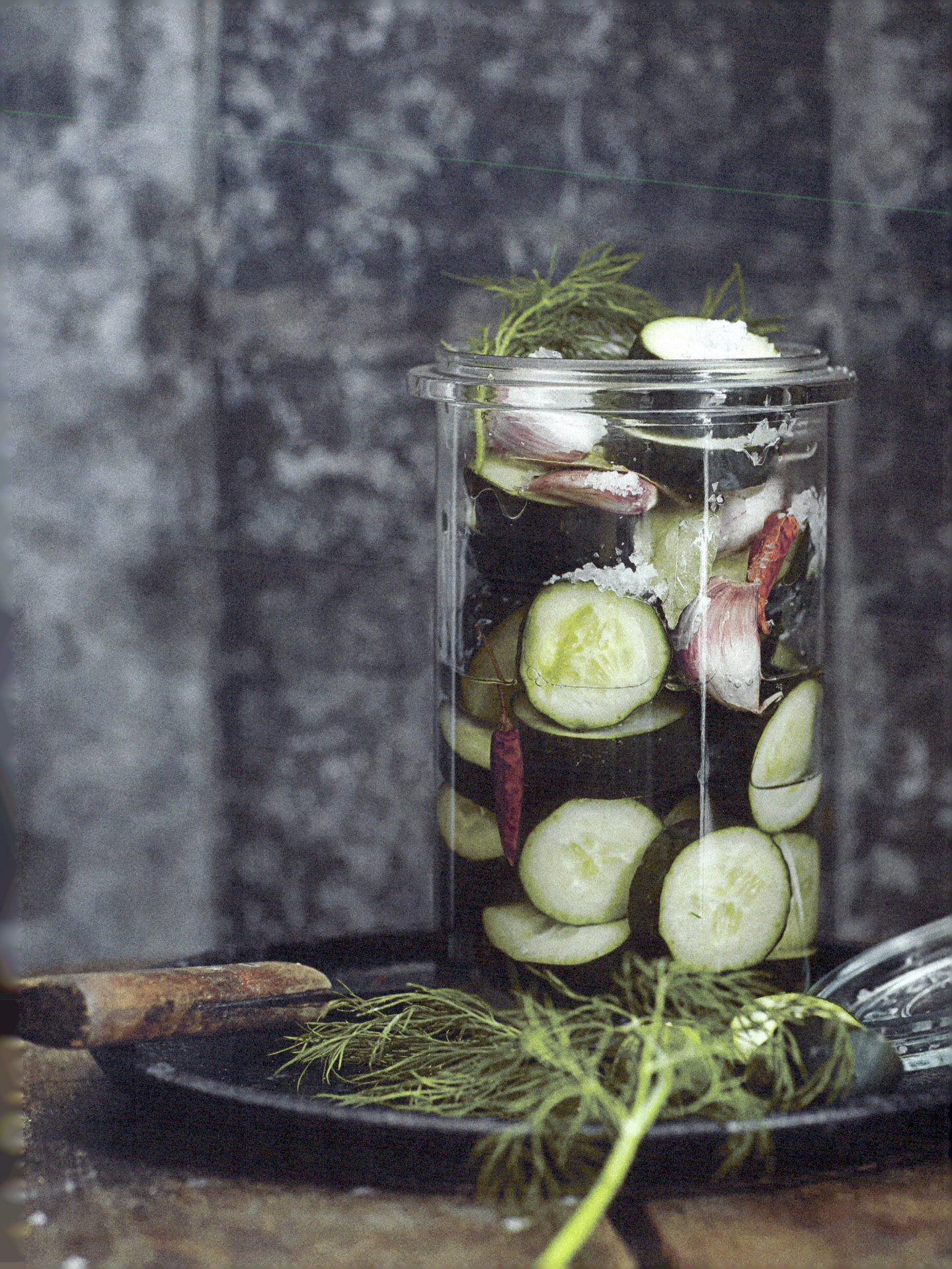

KASIA LEONARDI,
Krakow

CUISINE BETWEEN TWO WORLDS

It wasn't until she was in her mid-twenties that Kasia Leonardi found out about her Jewish origins. Since then, a lot has taken place for the Krakow native. Along with her sister, she has not only read up on her family history, but she has also completed a Conservative conversion, and married a New York City native of Jewish descent. In her personal journey back to her Jewish roots, food has played an important role. Not long after finding out about their Jewish past, Kasia and her sister began participating in events with the Jewish community in Krakow and, as part of that, they began cooking with them for Sabbat. In the Jewish community, she began to connect her Polish and Jewish roots through food; she quickly realized that Jewish Ashkenazi cuisine shared a lot of similarities with that of her Polish grandmother's, which made it seem familiar.

Merging these two strands of her heritage through food was natural fit for Kasia. She comes from a long line of epicureans. Her grandmother grew up in what is now a part of the Ukraine. Even so, her cooking was mostly influenced by Polish cuisine and by her desire to experiment with tastes and recipes that originated outside of Krakow. She liked to stress the acidic flavors in her cooking and undertook a lot of pickling. She taught Kasia how to pickle vegetables and make dumplings. When she thinks of her grandmother, Kasia makes mushroom dumplings and borscht; pickles her own red beets; and then uses the juice to make soup. From her Polish grandfather, from Poznan, she inherited an appreciation for the sweeter side of Polish cuisine.

Food continues to be bound up with Kasia's personal and professional life. She has become the official cook for the Jewish community in Krakow and travels extensively in Europe doing educational work on Polish-Jewish cuisine. In her travels, she tries to learn more about the culture at each place through its regional cuisine. She is especially interested in how food can bridge borders.

Kasia's cooking is lighter and more modern than the traditional, heavy Jewish-Polish cuisine. She tries to combine traditional Polish cuisine with modern Israeli cuisine for Krakow's Jewish community. She enjoys surprising its members with falafel, hummus, pita or baba ghanoush. She serves them alongside—what else?—none other than dumplings, just like her grandmother made.

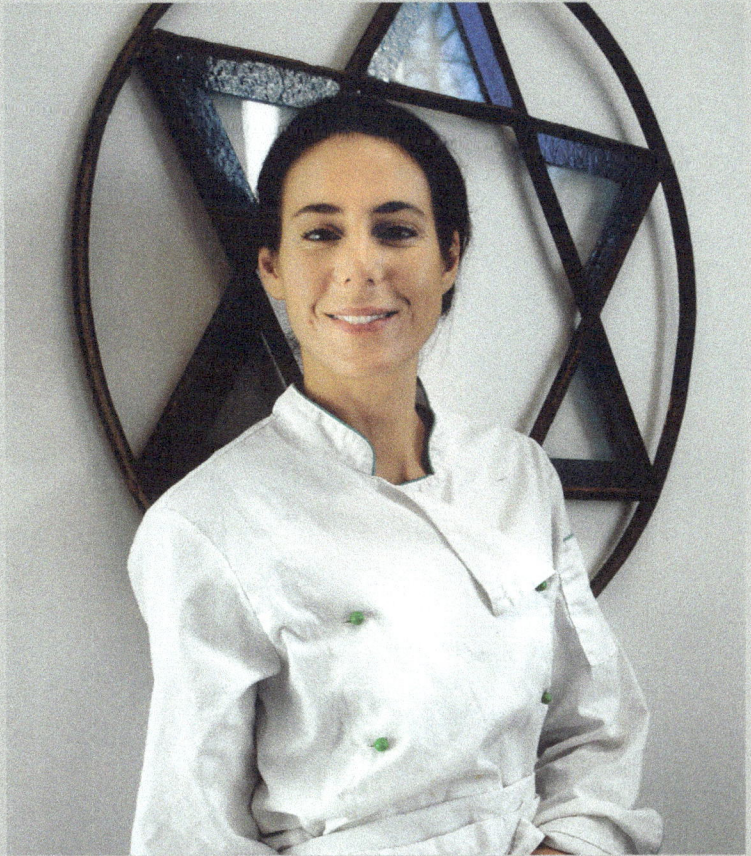

Kasia Leonardi didn't know about her Jewish origins for a long time. But she's been cooking her way through her cultural heritage ever since.

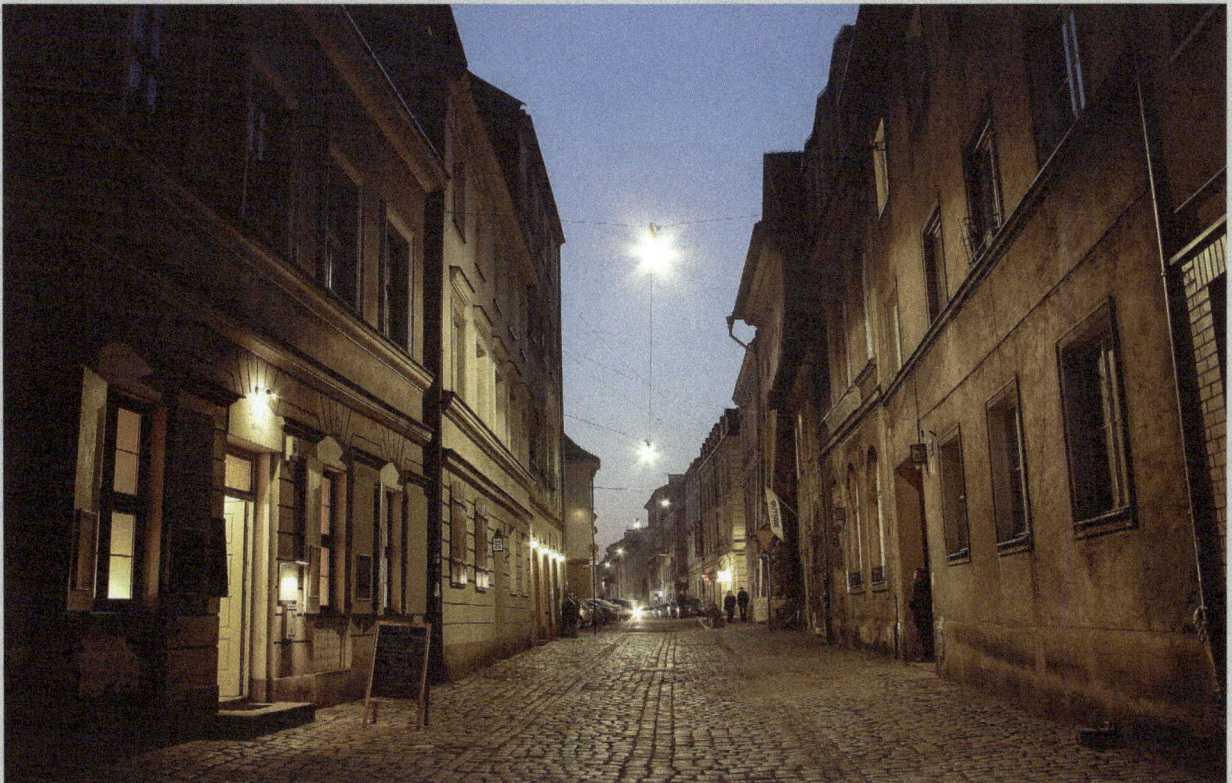

BORSCHT

BORSCHT
½ oz (5 g) dried
   mushrooms (such as,
   champignons, porcini)
1 lb (500 g) beets, about
   3-4 medium beets
1 bay leaf
2 pimento seeds
2 cups (500 mL) juice of
   pickled beet (see recipe
   on p. 142)
Salt
Sugar
Freshly ground black
   pepper

BORSCHT

1. Scald the dried mushrooms with 1 cup of boiling water, cover and let soak for about 1 hour.
2. Clean the beets thoroughly with a vegetable brush and water and place unpeeled in a pot. Add the bay leaf and allspice seeds. Then pour in 4 cups of water so that everything is covered. Bring to a boil and cook the beets until fork tender.
3. Remove the cooked beets from the water. Set the cooking water aside. Drain the soaked mushrooms but save the water in a bowl. Add the mushroom water and the juice from the beets to the beetroot cooking water and return to a boil.
4. Peel the cooked beets, cut into bite-sized pieces or grate coarsely and return to the pot. Coarsely chop the soaked mushrooms, if desired, and add to the pot as well. (Alternatively, use the mushrooms as a filling for uszka, see recipe on p. 144.)
5. Finally, season the soup with salt, sugar, and freshly ground pepper.

TO SERVE
Divide the borscht among 4 bowls and serve hot.

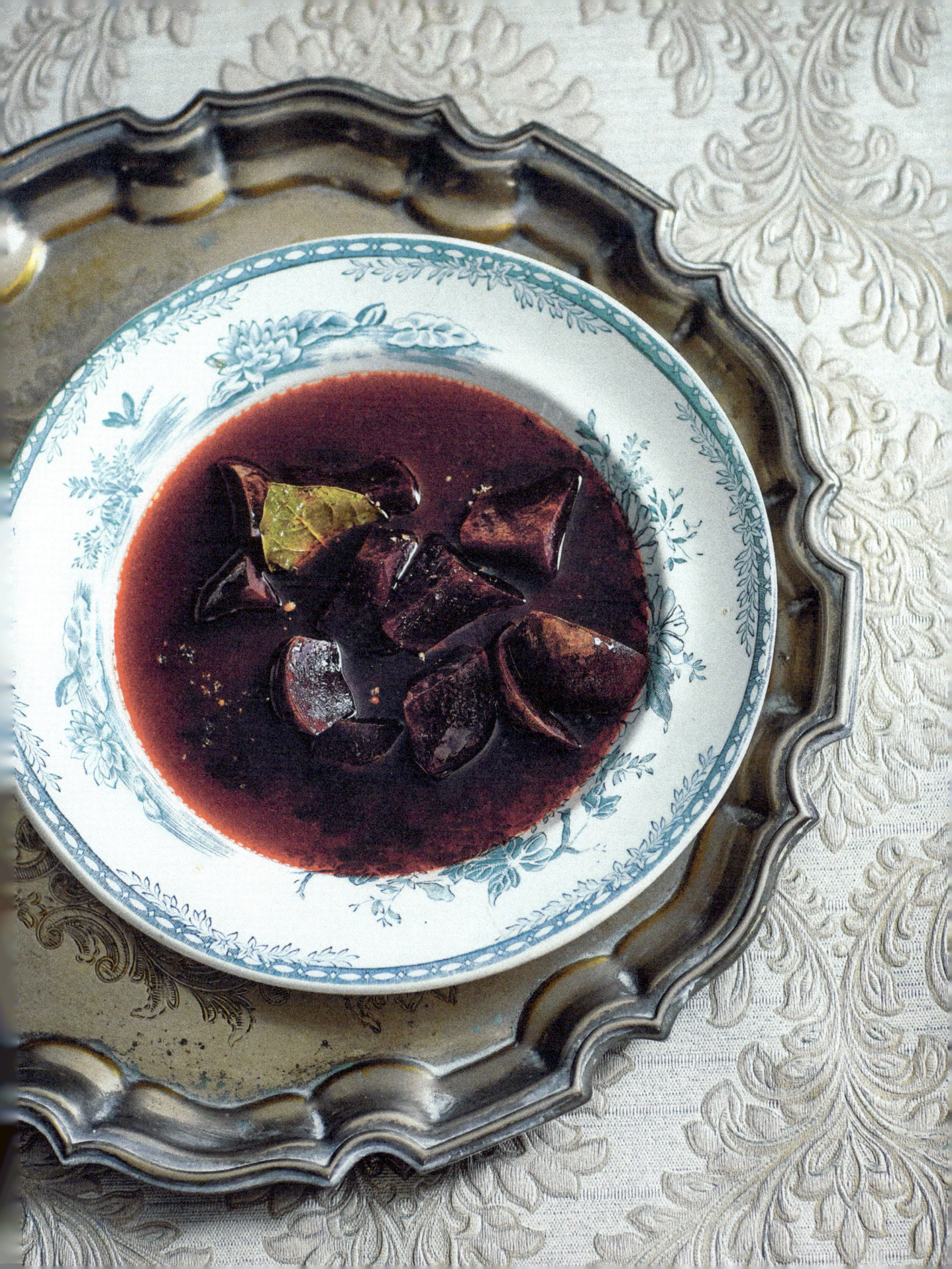

PICKLED RED-BEET JUICE

MAKES ABOUT 1-3 quarts
  (1-3 L)
PREPARATION: 20 MIN.
TO INFUSE: 5-7 DAYS

PICKLED RED-BEET JUICE
3 1/3 lb (1.5 kg) beets
3 cloves of garlic
½ tablespoon yellow mustard
seeds, to taste
6 cups (1.5 L) water
2 tablespoons salt

PICKLED RED-BEET JUICE

1. Wash the beets thoroughly with a vegetable brush, removing soil and sand. Then cut into thick slices or coarse pieces and place in one large or several smaller canning jars. Peel the garlic cloves, crush them with the blade of a knife and distribute them in the jars. Add yellow mustard seeds if desired.
2. Bring the water to the boil with the salt until the salt is completely dissolved. Let the stock cool, then pour into the prepared jars so that the vegetables are fully covered. Add additional water as needed.
3. Close the jars tightly and leave to infuse in a cool, dark place or in the refrigerator for 5-7 days.
4. Strain the juice before use. This juice can be used for borscht (see recipe on p. 140).144.)
5. Finally, season the soup with salt, sugar, and freshly ground pepper.

TO SERVE
Divide the borscht among 4 bowls and serve hot.

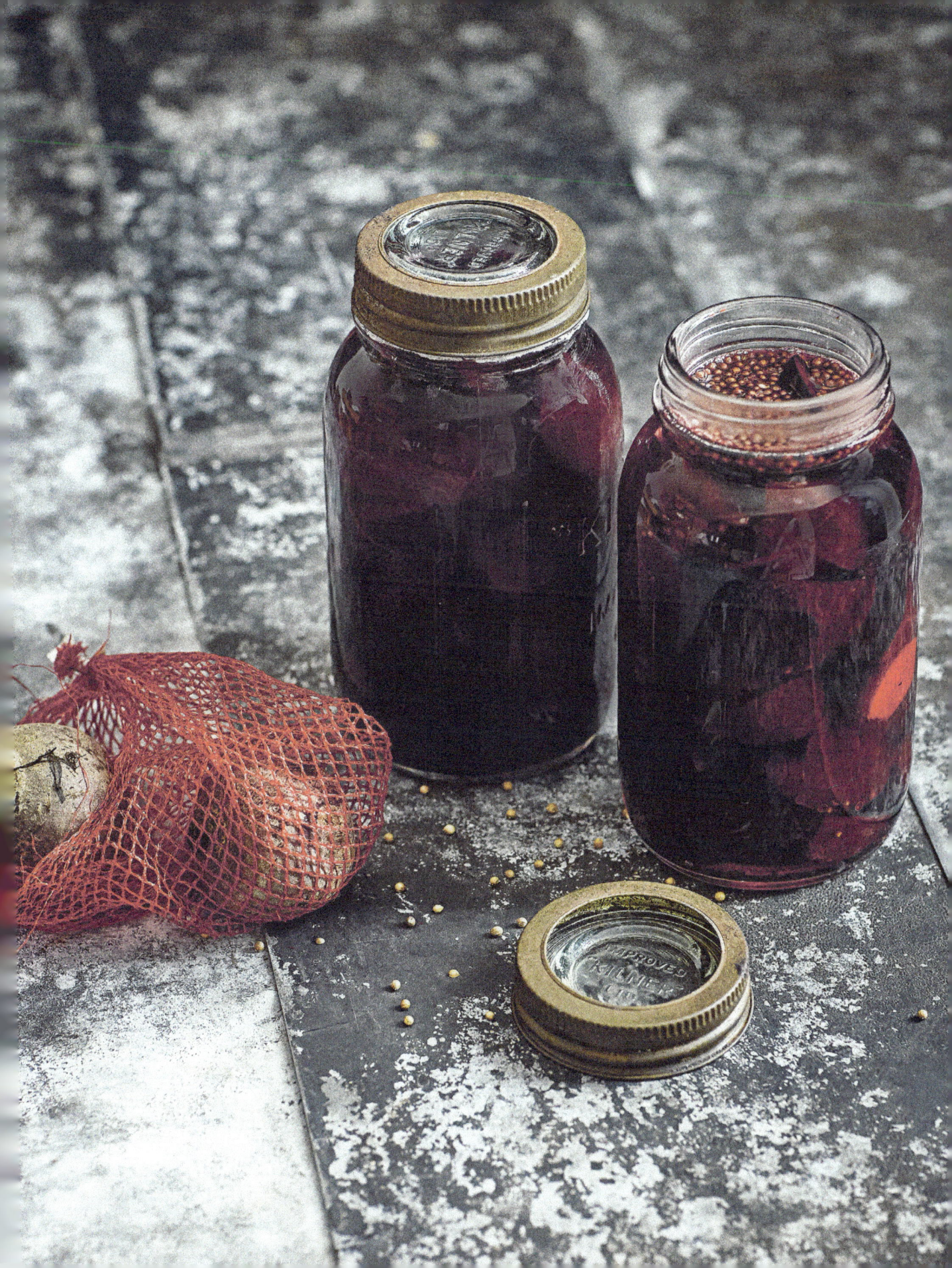

USZKA
—MUSHROOM DUMPLINGS

SERVES 4/ MAKES ABOUT
    18-20 USZKAS
PREPARATION: 50 MIN.
SOAKING TIME: 12 HRS.

MUSHROOM FILLING
1 oz (20 g) dried
    mushrooms (mixed
    forest mushrooms,
    porcini or morels)
1 onion (80 g)
1 tablespoon butter
1 tablespoon breadcrumbs
Salt
Freshly ground black
    pepper

USZKA
2 eggs
1 cup (240 mL) boiling
    water
1 2/3 cups (240 g) all-
    purpose flour, plus
    some for adding to
    mushroom filling
Salt
1 tablespoon vegetable oil

MUSHROOM FILLING

1. Put the dried mushrooms in a heat-resistant canning jar and cover with boiling water. Close the jar and soak the mushrooms for about 12 hours.
2. Peel and dice the onion. Melt the butter in a pan and sweat the onions until translucent. Remove the mushrooms from the soaking water, add to the onions and cook for 1 minute. Strain the leftover mushroom soaking water through a fine-mesh sieve and set aside. Place the entire contents of the pan, plus the breadcrumbs, in a small food processor and coarsely blend. Season the mushroom filling with salt and freshly ground pepper and allow to cool.

USZKA

1. Separate the eggs and place the whites and yolks in separate bowls. In another bowl, whisk together the boiling water, half of the flour, and 1 large pinch of salt until no large lumps remain. Add the remaining flour and knead everything together on a work surface. Add the vegetable oil and the egg yolks one at a time until the dough is elastic and easy to shape.

FINAL STEPS

4 cups (1 L) chicken stock
   (see recipe
   p. 120)
Mushroom soaking water
Salt
Freshly ground black
   pepper
4 tablespoons sour cream
Some freshly grated
   horseradish
Celery stalks

2. Onto a lightly floured surface, roll out the dough into a 1/8-inch-thin rectangle and cut out squares, about 3 x 3 inches. Put 2 teaspoons of mushroom filling in the center of each square. Brush the edges with a little egg white and fold into a triangle. Brush the two corners of the dough with a little egg white, fold over each other and press together.

FINAL STEPS

1. Bring the chicken stock and the strained mushroom soaking water to a boil in a saucepan. Add the uszkas and cook for 5-8 minutes until they rise to the top of the water. Season the chicken stock with salt and freshly ground pepper to taste.
2. Serve the uszkas with the chicken stock and top with some sour cream, fresh horseradish, and celery.

Tip: The uszkas also taste great with borscht (see recipe on p. 140). You can simply cook the dumplings ahead of time in a pot of gently boiling water.

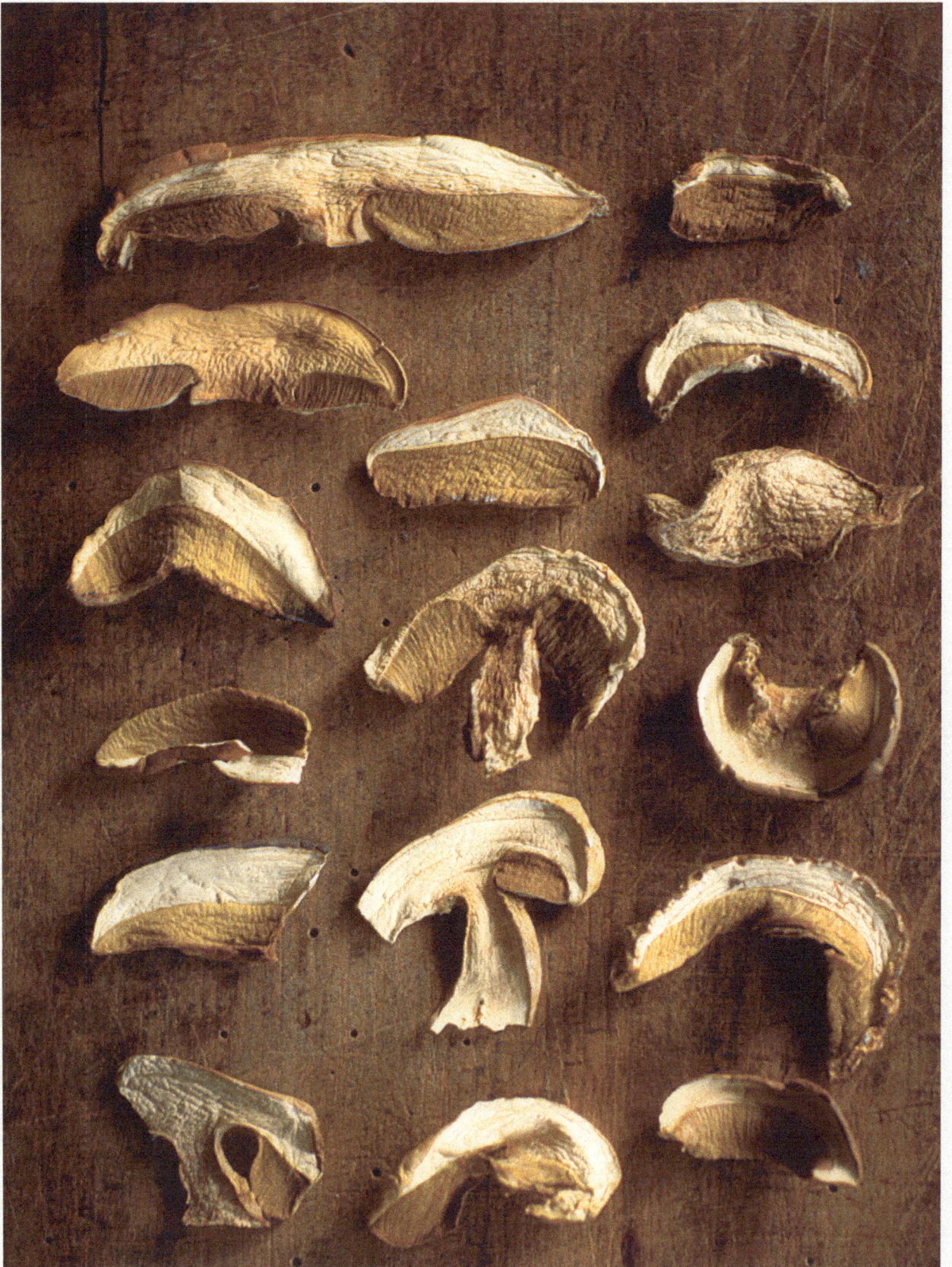

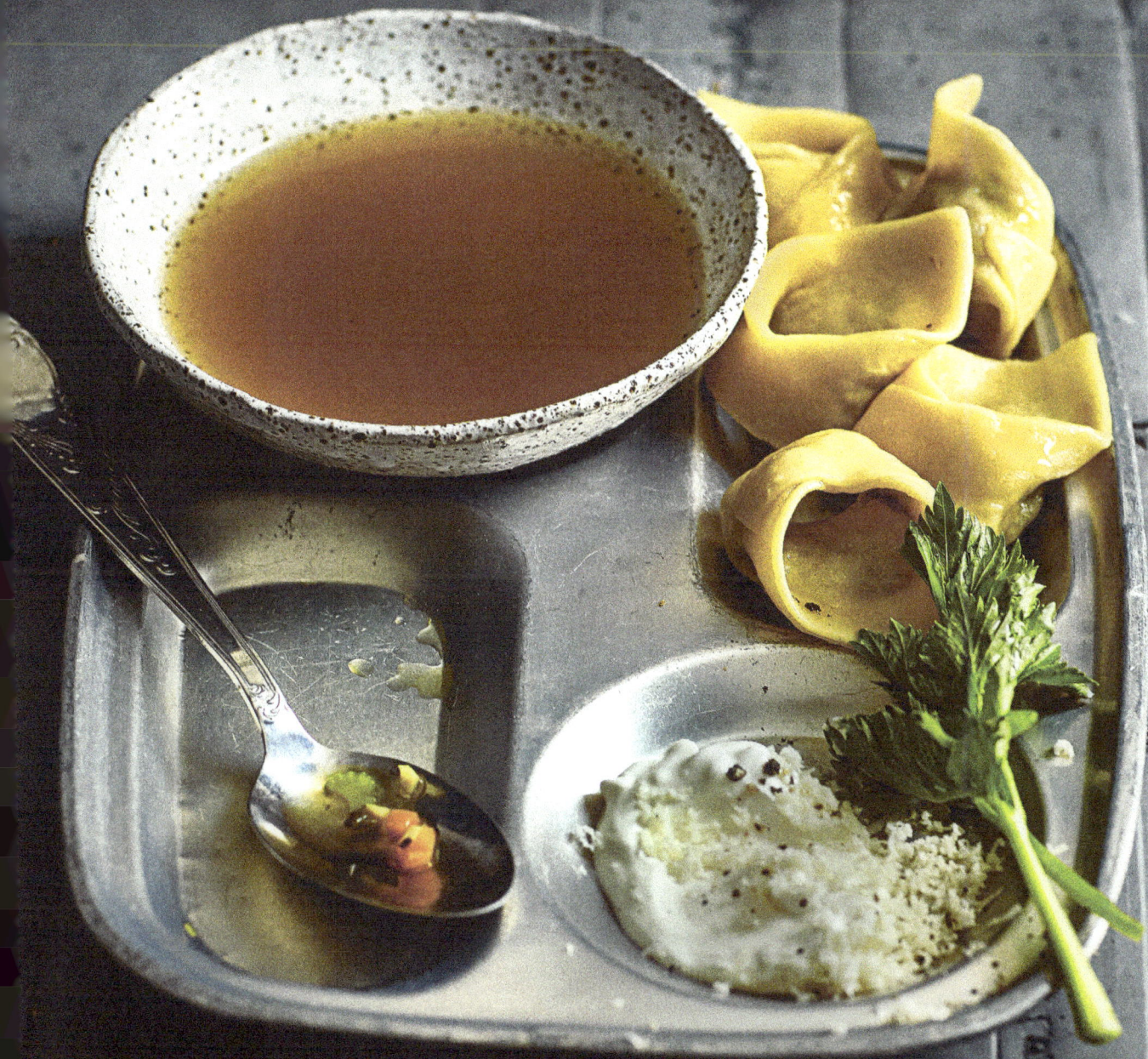

POPPY SEED STRUDEL

SERVES 4- 6 / MAKES 2 STRUDELS
PREPARATION TIME: 40 MIN.
RISING TIME: 1 ¼-1 ¾ HRS.
BAKING TIME: 40-50 MIN.

DOUGH
3 cups (360 g) either pastry or all-purpose
   flour
4 ½ teaspoons (15 g) active dry yeast
¾ cup (180 mL) milk, lukewarm
6 egg yolks
6 tablespoons sugar
½ teaspoon salt
2 tablespoons rum or almond liqueur
2 teaspoons vanilla extract
11 tablespoons (150 g) butter, melted

POPPY SEED FILLING
1 ½ cups (250 g) poppy seeds
½ cups (90 g) brown sugar
¼ cup (50 g) raisins
¼ cup (25 g) walnuts
3 tablespoons honey
2 drops of almond extract
1 teaspoon butter
3/4 cup (60 g) candied orange peel
6 egg whites

FINAL STEPS
Flour for work surface
1 egg
2 tablespoons milk

DOUGH
1. Mix the flour with the dry yeast in a large bowl. Add the lukewarm milk, the egg yolks, the sugar, the salt, the rum or liqueur, and the vanilla extract and knead everything together. Add the melted butter and knead until a shiny, smooth dough is formed. Transfer the dough to the lightly floured work surface and shape into a ball.
2. Put the dough back in the bowl, cover and let rise in a warm, dark place for 1-1½ hours until it has doubled in size.

POPPY SEED FILLING
1. Remove 4 tablespoons of poppy seeds and set aside for sprinkling later. Place the remaining poppy seeds in a bowl, scald with boiling water and set aside.
2. When the scalded poppy seeds have reached room temperature, drain, and finely grind in a blender. Add the brown sugar, raisins, walnuts, honey, almond extract, butter, and candied orange peel and blend well. Pour the poppy seed mixture into a bowl and stir in the egg whites.

FINAL STEPS
1. Preheat the oven to 350°F. Line a baking sheet with parchment paper.
2. Divide the dough into 2 equal pieces, roll them out evenly into rectangles and spread with the poppy seed filling. Leave a 3/4-inch margin all around. Roll up the dough, fold in the ends and place on the baking sheet.
3. Whisk the egg and milk and brush the strudels with it. Sprinkle with the remaining poppy seeds and let rest for 15 minutes. Bake for 40-50 minutes until golden brown.
4. Allow to cool. Cut into slices before serving.

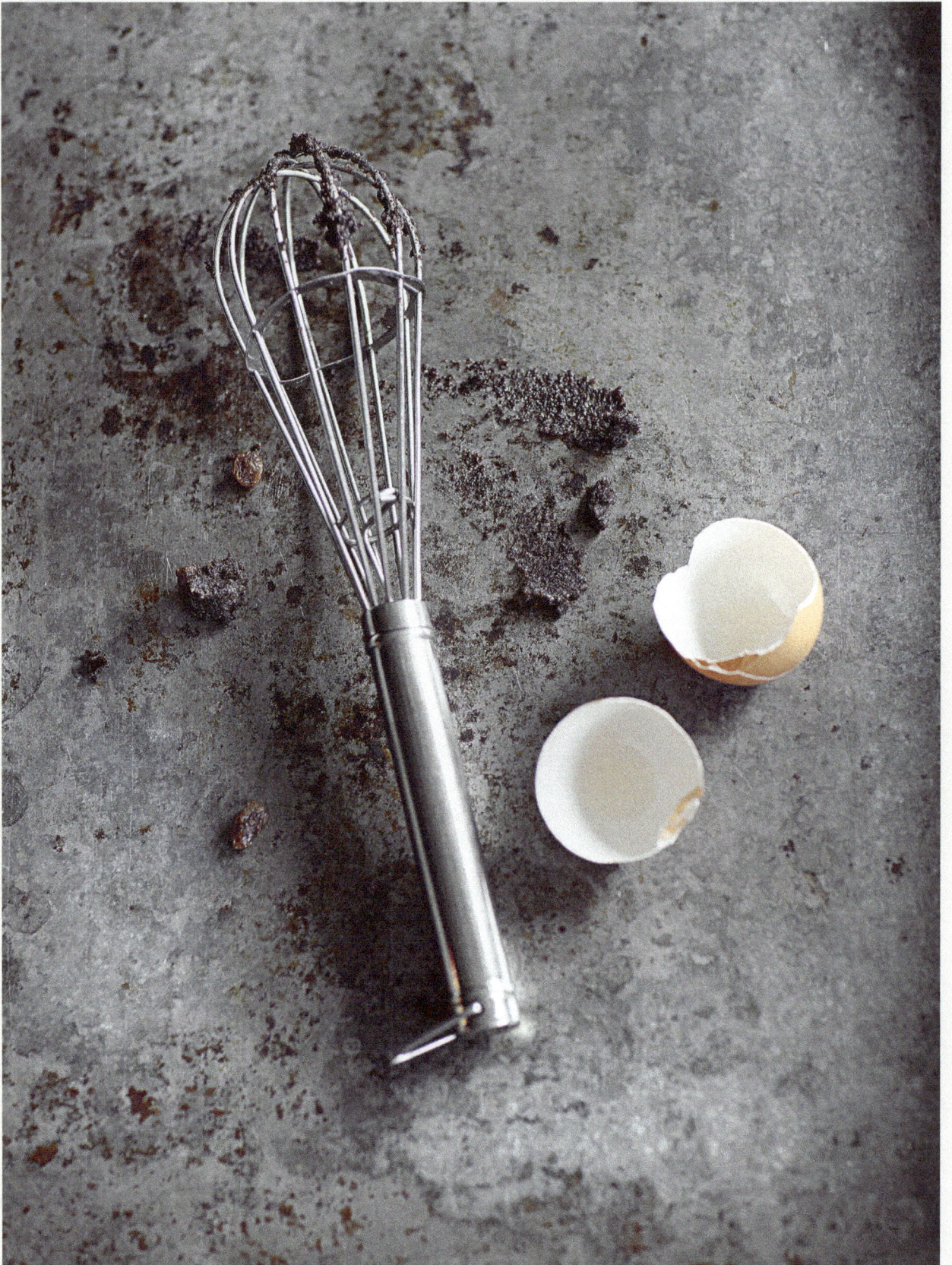

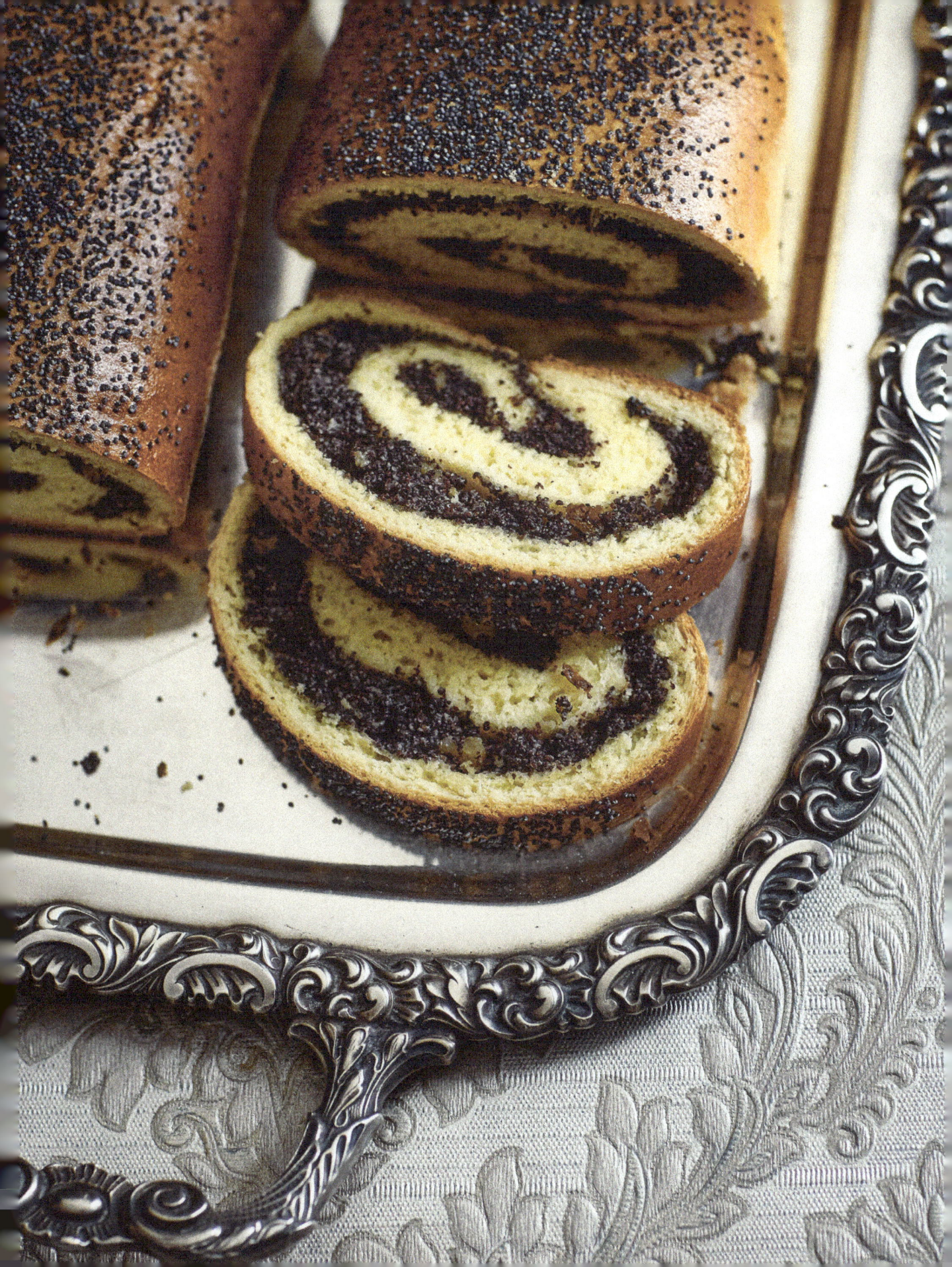

JACOB KENEDY, London

PREPARED WITH LOVE

Jacob Kenedy is one of London's most famous chefs. And he is one of the few chefs who actually grew up in London. But Jacob's parents came from elsewhere. His father has Jewish-Hungarian roots, but Jacob didn't know anything about his father's history until he was 18. What he found out was that during the Second World War his father's family had fled to Ireland and changed their last name to hide the fact that they were Jewish. Jacob's mother grew up in Italy and lived in Austria before moving to London. His family's history has been a rich source of influences on which he has drawn.

Included among those sources of inspiration are his mother's and especially his grandmothers' cooking. From his mother, he inherited a love for a chicken soup made to suit your mood or the ingredients that you have on hand. As he explains, "When I am feeling ill or mum is, or she is happy or depressed, or lonely or in company, she makes chicken soup. It's different every time but always tastes recognisably hers, seasoned with love and warmth and affection." One of Jacob's favorite dishes, rakott káposzta, comes from his Hungarian-Jewish side. It's a casserole dish with less than kosher ingredients. Topped with sauerkraut, yogurt, and sour cream, it includes not only a pound-and-a-half of minced pork but also various Hungarian kolbás sausages. A truly hearty dish! From the other side of his family, Jacob adores his Italian grandmother Agnes' doughnuts. He has served them in every restaurant in which he has ever worked. It's hard to argue with the pleasure

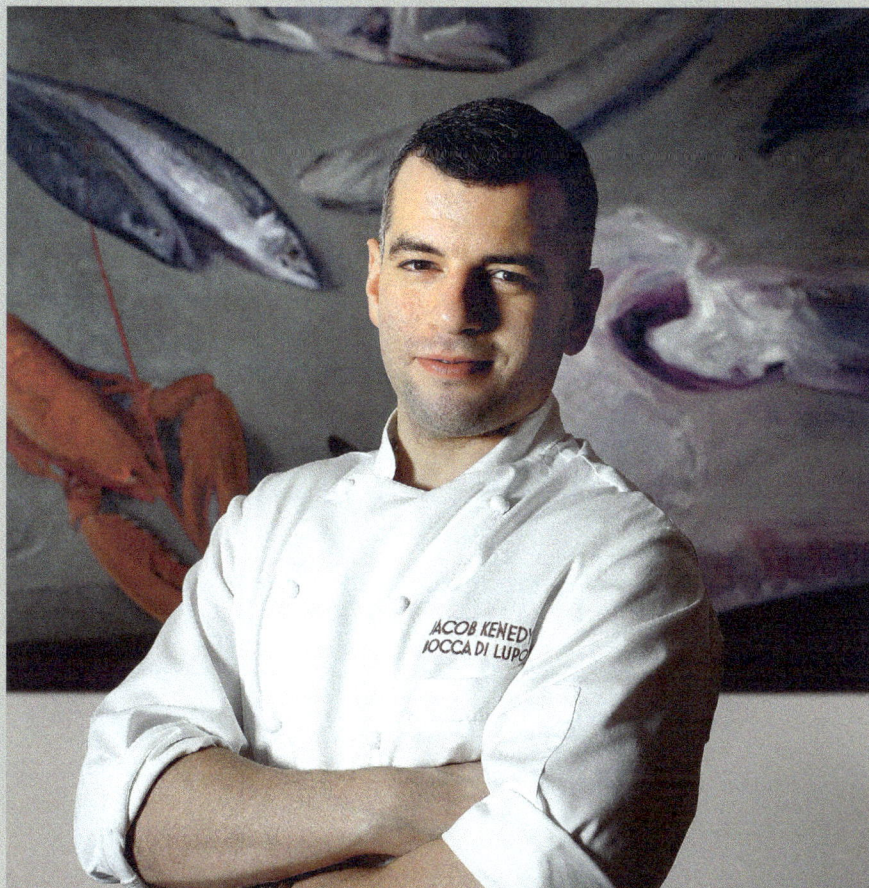

His Italian roots have influenced him throughout his life. He is especially well known for his chocolate-filled doughnuts.

of deep-fried dough filled with chocolate cream, in whatever way shape or form it may come. But Jacob claims that his recipe is the best! He got from his grandmother after all. The bombe calde (Italian for filled doughnuts) are popular with adults and kids alike. What makes Jacob's recipe so special is that the doughnuts are filled with more "chocolate cream than is good for you." But they are not too sweet; the recipe calls for only a small amount of sugar in the chocolate cream filling.

Jewish tradition, of course, also shaped Jacob's relationship to cooking. He didn't grow up in a religious household, but his family made a big fuss over the holidays. And Jacob's mother always expressed an appreciation for the role that the table plays in Jewish culture. She taught him about its importance when he was still young and learning, in her words, to become a "fantastic eater."

For Jacob, Jewish food means a mélange of different sources that may come from just about anywhere. It's steeped in history, something emotional, a story of survival, and above all else, it's linked with family. It's these ties to Jewish tradition and history, that inspire people to pay more attention to the background connected to traditional Jewish recipes and to feel connected to their preparation. People, he observes, tend to cook dishes better when the dish has personal meaning to them. That's how he works, too. At the end of the day, he says, it has to do with love. When something is prepared with love, it tastes good.

MUM'S CHICKEN SOUP

SERVES 4
PREPARATION: 30 MIN.
COOKING TIME: 1 ½ HRS.

CHICKEN STOCK
1 (2-3 lb) whole, free roaming
   chicken
5 cloves garlic, halved

Your Choice
2-4 of the following:
   1 leek, 3 stalks celery, parsnip
   carrot, onion, or fennel
1 or more of the following:
   2 bay leaves, 1 teaspoon
   peppercorns, 1 teaspoon fennel
   seeds, 1 chipotle or ancho
   chile, 1-inch fresh turmeric,
   1-inch fresh ginger

CHICKEN STOCK
1. Rinse the chicken under cold running water.
Place in a large pot, covering generously with cold
water.
2. Depending on which 2-3 vegetables you choose:
clean, peel, coarsely chop and add to the pot along
with the garlic and chosen spices.
3. Bring to a slow boil, reduce heat, and allow to
simmer for 1 hour, skimming off the foam with a
ladle or spoon.
 4. When chicken is almost falling off the bone,
remove from the pot and strain the stock. Set aside
1 cup and put the rest back into the pot. Pick the
chicken meat off the bones, discarding the skin.
Shred half of the meat and put back in the pot with
the stock. Reserve the other half of the meat for an
alternate use. Season with salt and freshly ground
pepper.

SOUP

Your Choice

1-3 of the following:
  1 leek, 2 carrots, 2 stalks celery, 1 wedge pumpkin or other starchy squash, 1 quarter celeriac

1 of the following:
  1, 4.5 oz matzo ball mix, make per pack instructions and roll into mini ½-inch balls, 5 oz (150g) dried egg pappardelle, broken into bite-sized pieces, 3.5 oz (100g) orzo pasta, 3 oz (80g) barley or rice

3 tablespoons chopped parsley

1 of the following:
  juice of 1 lemon or 2 limes, ¼ red onion, chopped & mixed with 4 tablespoons red wine vinegar, 2 large gherkins, chopped, plus 4 tablespoons gherkin pickling juice

Salt

Freshly ground black pepper

SOUP

1. Cook chosen starch according to directions on the package, using the reserved ½ cup chicken stock for added flavor. Be careful not to overcook.

2. Wash, peel, and dice chosen vegetables into bite-sized pieces and add to the pot with chicken and stock. Bring to a low boil and simmer for 15 minutes or until vegetables are soft.

3. Just before serving, add the cooked starch, chopped parsley, and the chosen acid (lemon, lime, gherkin, or red onion) and stir everything together. Add salt and freshly ground black pepper to taste.

TO SERVE

Divide the soup among 4 bowls and serve hot.

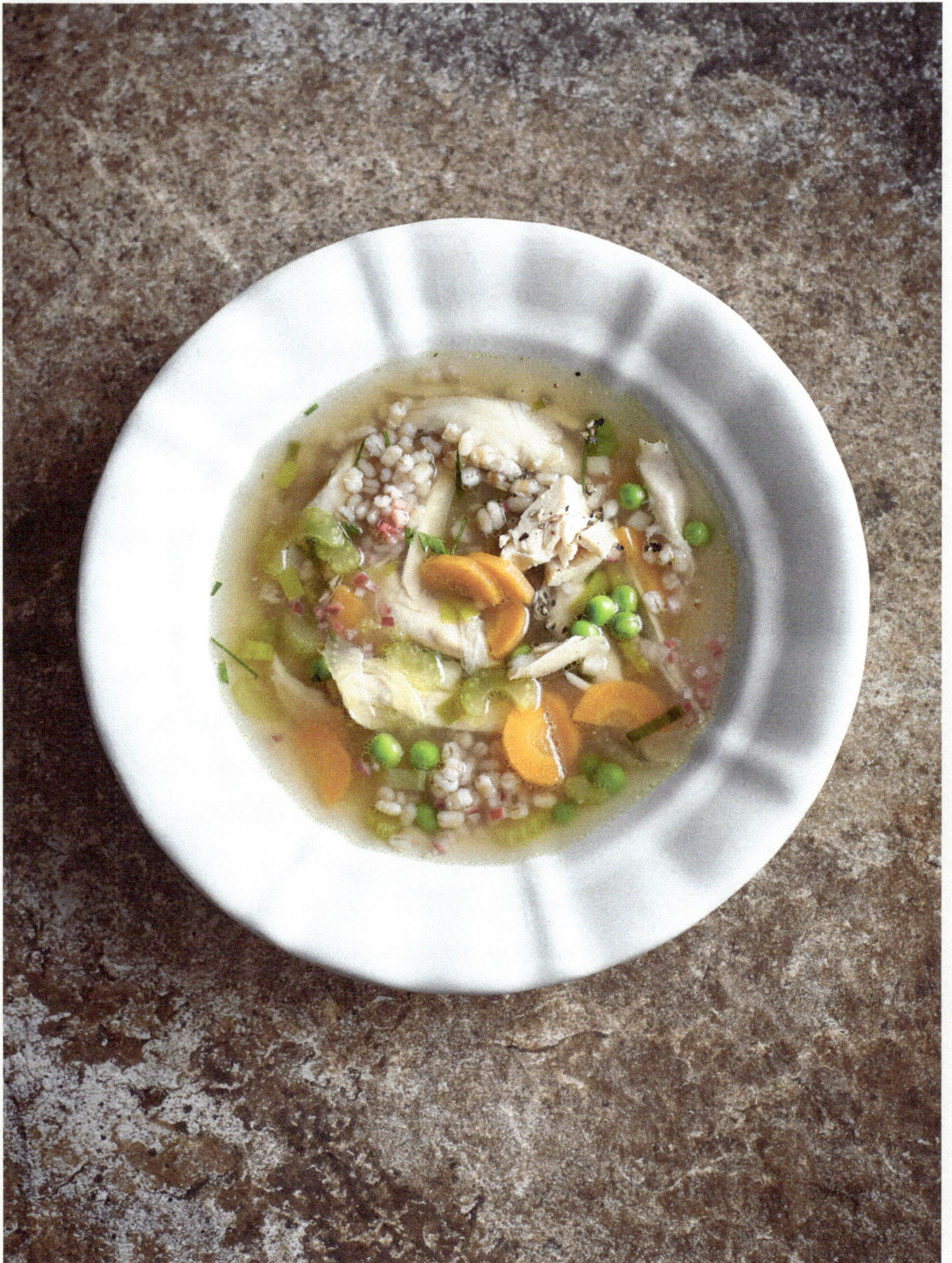

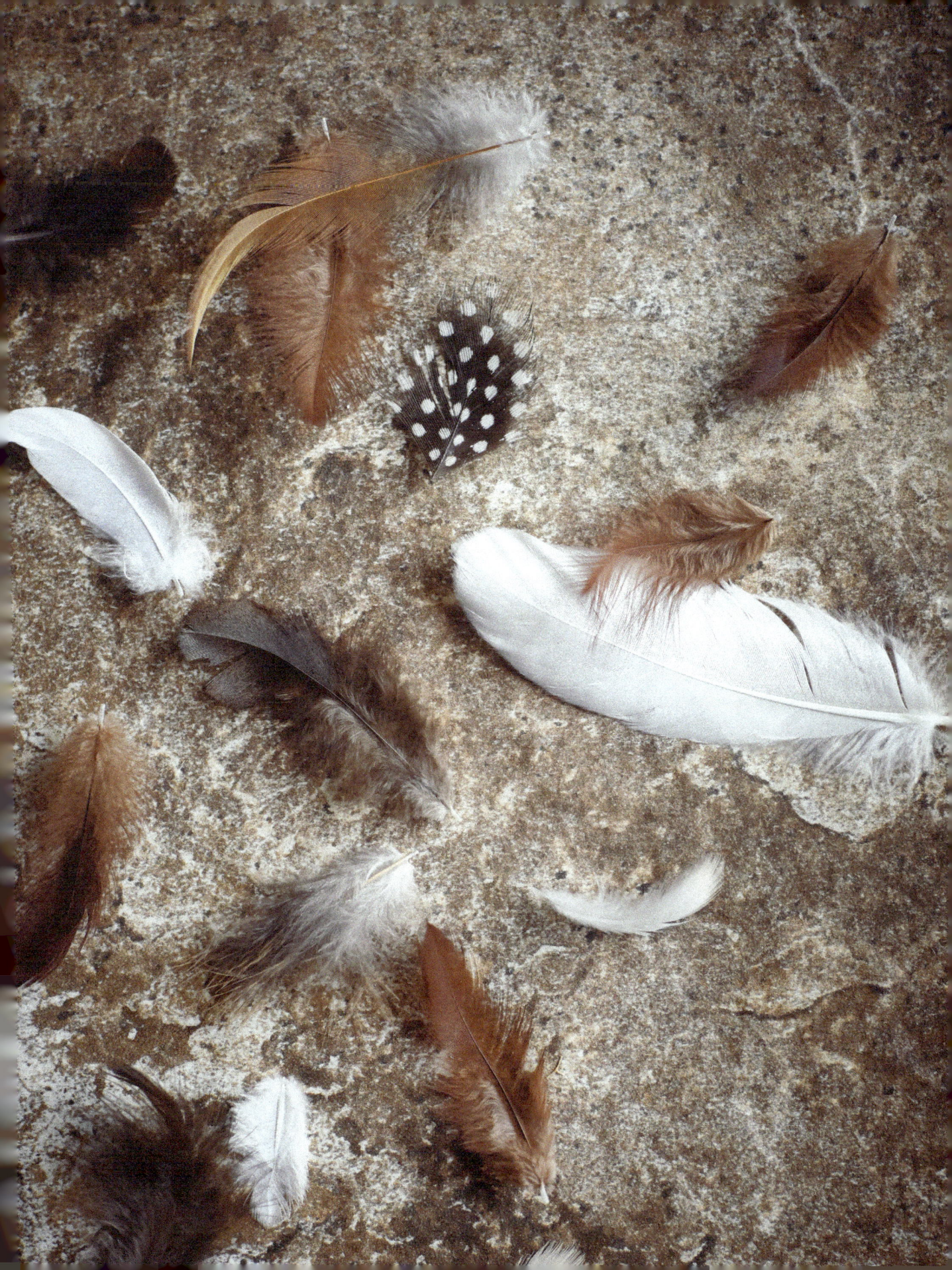

GRANDMA AGNES' DOUGHNUTS

MAKES 12-14 LARGE DOUGHNUTS
PREPARATION TIME: 3 ½ HRS.
RISING TIME: 2 HRS.
FRYING TIME & LAST STEPS: 30 MIN.

DOUGH
3 ½ teaspoons (10 g) active dry yeast
1 1/3 cups (280 mL) milk, lukewarm
4 ½ cups (560 g) all-purpose flour
¼ cup (50 g) caster sugar
Pinch of salt
8 large egg yolks
2 tablespoons dark rum
Zest of 1 lemon, grated finely
7 tablespoons (100 g) unsalted butter, melted

FILLING
1 cup (200 mL) heavy cream
4 large egg yolks
½ cup (50 g) cocoa powder
¾ cup (160 g) caster sugar
2 ½ tablespoons (20 g) corn flour
2 cups (500 mL) milk
1 cinnamon stick
4 ½ oz (120 g) bittersweet chocolate, broken
   into pieces

TO COOK AND SERVE
Vegetable oil
Powdered sugar

DOUGH

1. Start making the dough about 3 hours before you wish to fry and serve the doughnuts. First make a yeast sponge. In a small bowl, mix the yeast with half of the milk and a tablespoon each of the flour and sugar. Leave to rise until frothy.

2. Mix the remaining flour and sugar with the salt in a large bowl, make a well in the middle and add the yeast sponge and all the other ingredients except the butter. Work in the flour gradually from the sides to make a sticky dough, which should be very well kneaded. When glossy and elastic, add the butter, gradually, and work until fully incorporated. Leave the dough to rise, covered, until doubled in size, just over an hour.

3. Roll the dough out ½-inch thick on a floured surface, and using a pastry cutter, cut them into rounds with about a 4-inch diameter. Dust very lightly with flour, cover with a light cloth, and leave to rise until doubled in size. About an hour.

FILLING

While the doughnuts are rising, make the filling. Whisk together the cream, egg yolks, cocoa, sugar, and corn flour to make a thick paste. In a small saucepan, add the cinnamon stick and milk and bring to a boil. Gradually add cinnamon-milk-mixture to the cocoa paste, whisking until fully incorporated. Return to the pan, and over the lowest flame, bring it to a gentle boil, stirring constantly with a wooden spoon or whisk. The mixture will thicken suddenly. As soon as it has boiled, take it off the heat, remove the cinnamon stick and add the chocolate, stirring continuously until it has melted. Transfer it to a squeeze bottle with a pointed nozzle and keep warm until ready to serve by standing the bottle up in a pan of hot water over very low heat.

TO COOK & SERVE

Heat at least 1 ½-inches of oil in a saucepan to 300°F. Fry the doughnuts, turning them once when the first side is golden, approximately 4 minutes on each side. When cooked all the way through, remove with tongs, and set onto paper towels to drain. Using the squeeze bottle, fill them with a generous amount of chocolate filling. Dust each bombe with powdered sugar and serve warm.

VARIATION: Dipping Doughnuts

Make the same dough but cut it into 2-inch rounds. Leave them to rise, then fry as above. Instead of filling them, serve them with a "jam dip" made with jam that has been warmed and thinned with a bit of water and accompanied by a generous pour of rum.

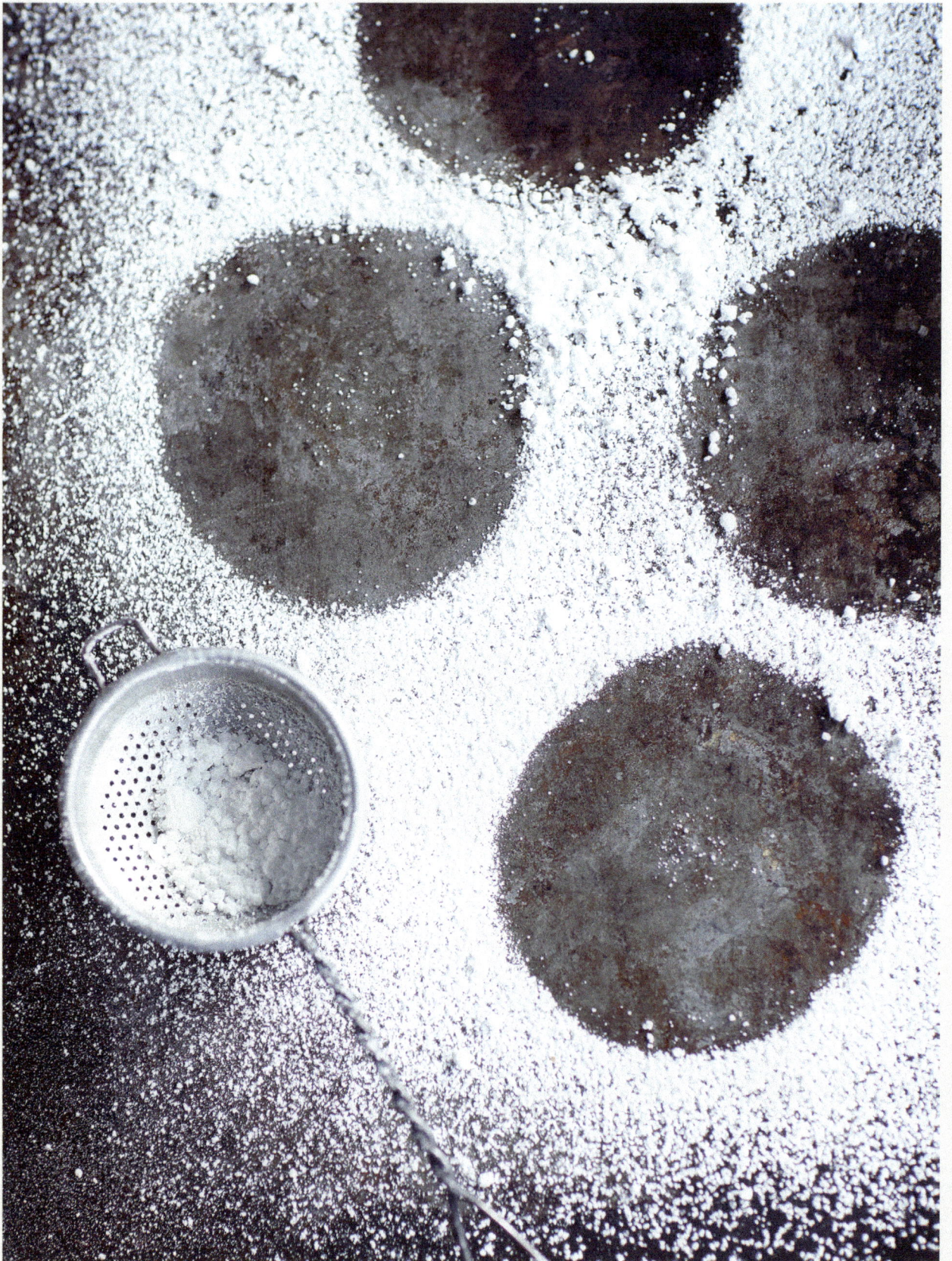

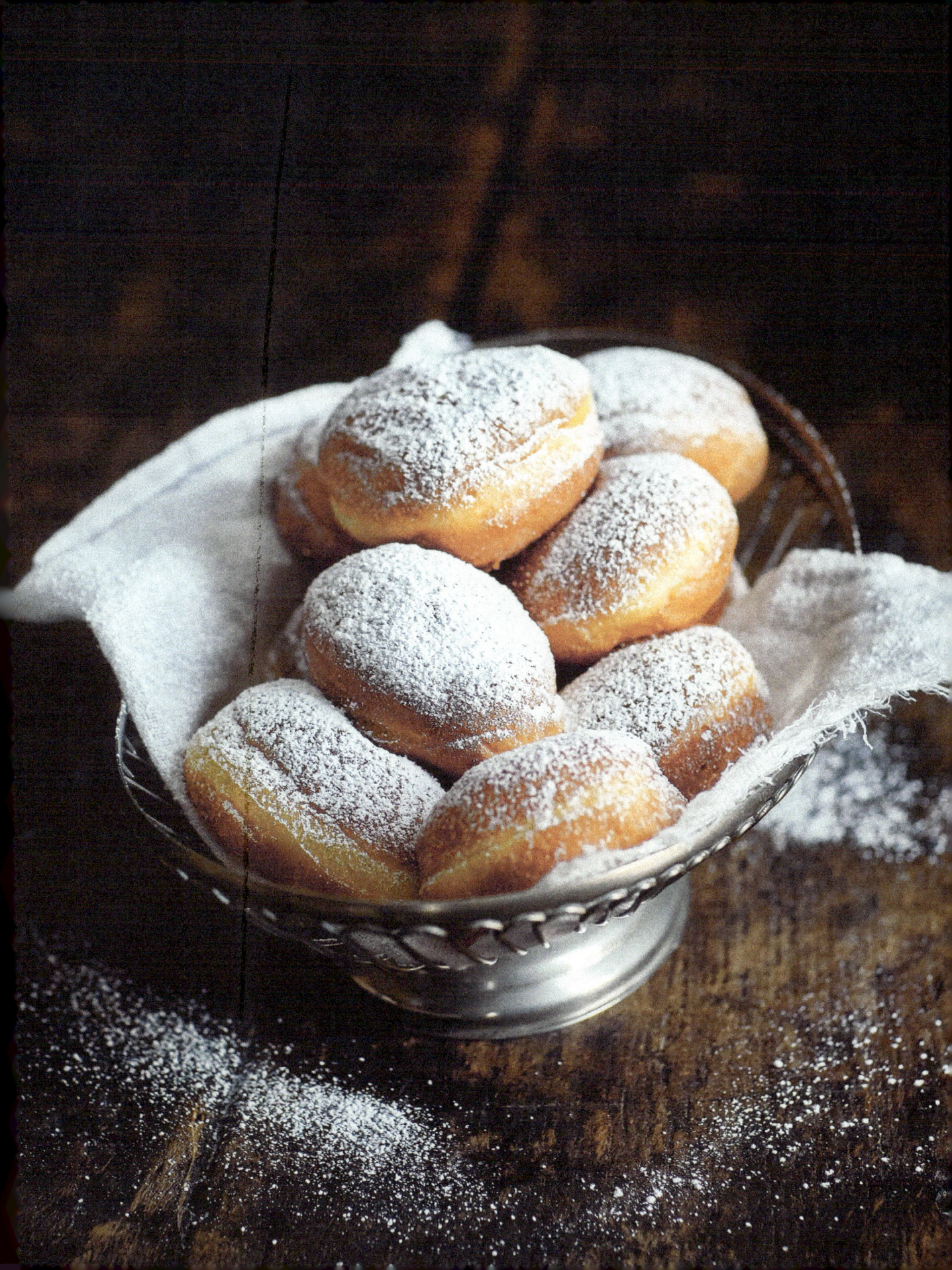

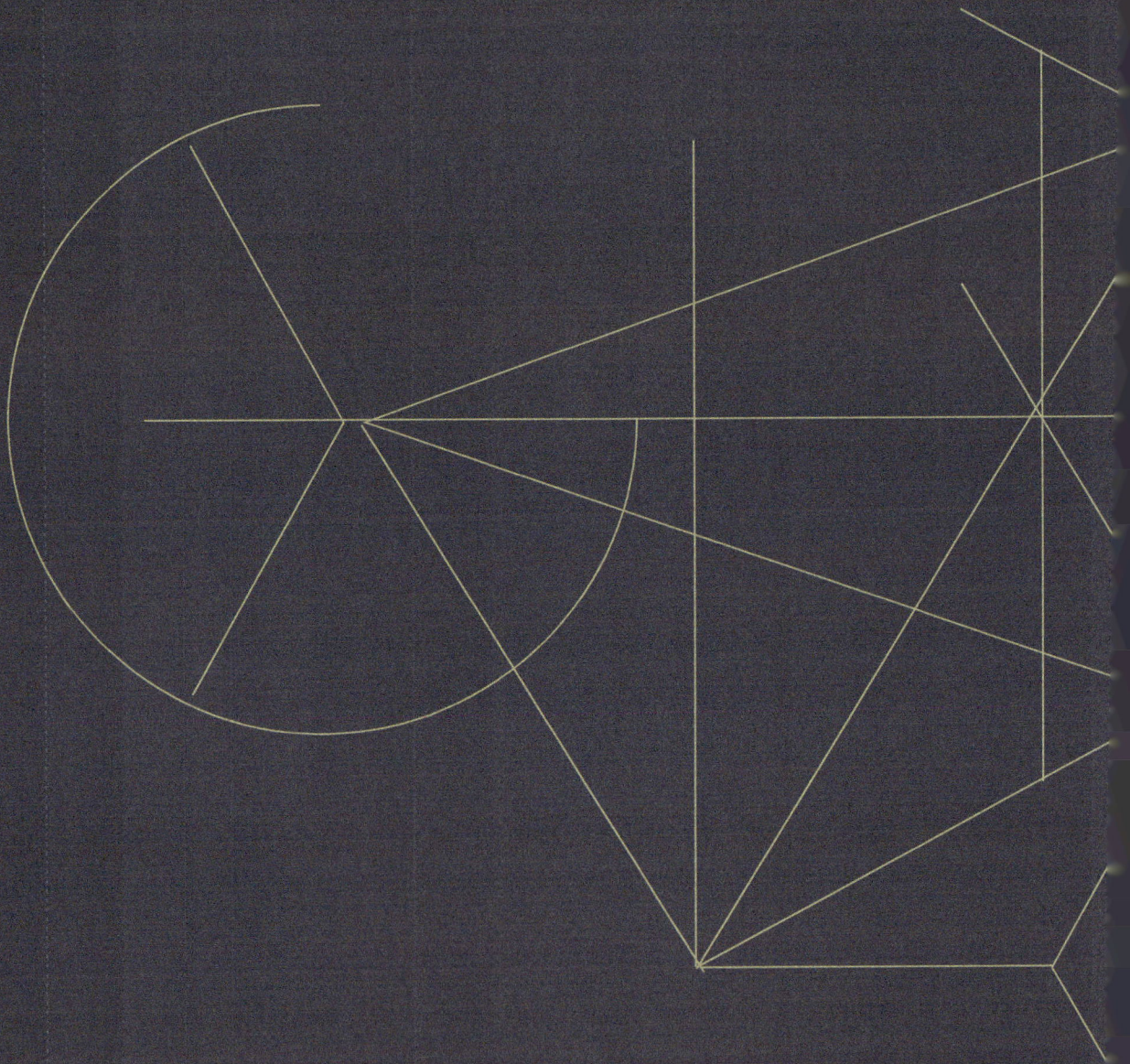

NEW

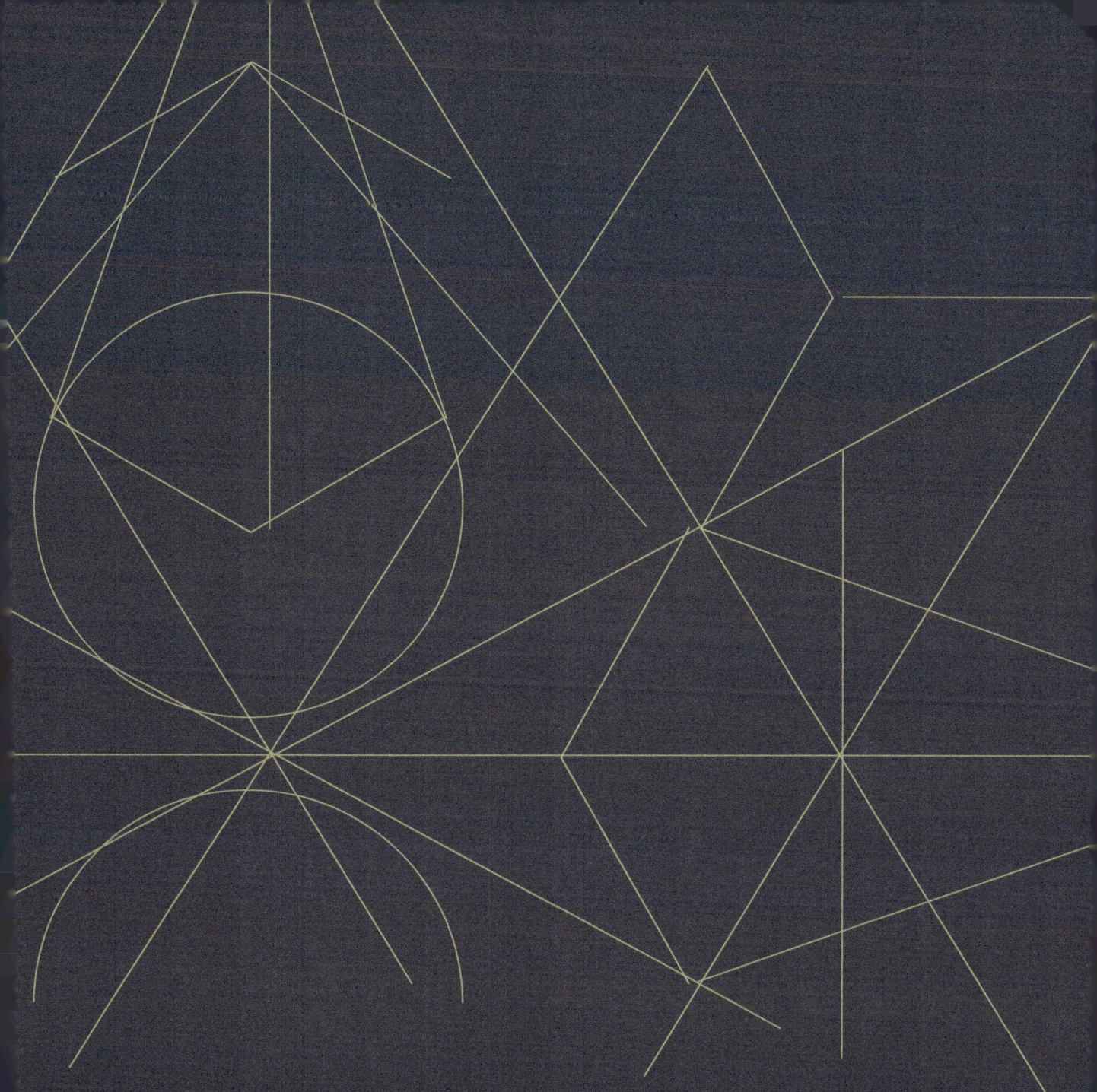

WORLD

LEAH KOENIG, New York

FOODIN THE AGE OF GLOBALIZAITON

If there is one person who can call herself an expert on global Jewish cuisine, it is Leah Koenig. Leah has been writing about the phenomenon of Jewish cuisine for years, and her work has been featured in publications such as the New York Times, the Wall Street Journal, Saveur, Epicurious, Food52, and Bon Appetit. She has also written several cookbooks, most recently The Jewish Cookbook that celebrates the diversity of Jewish cooking.

Leah learned to love cooking from her mother. Although they ate a lot of American food at home, they always had beef brisket, latkes, and challah at the holidays. It wasn't until college that Leah learned to cook for herself. She lovingly describes the food she prepared back then as "American hippie cuisine," lots of vegetable dishes, dark bread, and casseroles. But it made her realize that she had to cook for herself if she wanted to eat well.

Leah pursued a degree in Environmental Studies and Religion, and after college worked for the Jewish environmental organization Hazon, where she covered a mix of topics including Jewish tradition, agriculture, and sustainability. At the same time, she also started working as a journalist. She quickly realized that she could only become successful by writing about topics close to her heart. The more she became involved with Jewish cuisine, the more important it became for her to write about it from a broader perspective. That's why she started writing about global Jewish culture.

She is often surprised when she encounters a dish that somehow seems familiar, but that she herself has never actually made or even eaten before. One of her favorite examples is the cuisine of Ethiopian Jews. A few years ago, Leah cooked Doro Wat, an Ethiopian chicken stew with egg, with a friend, an Ethiopian-Jew. Doro

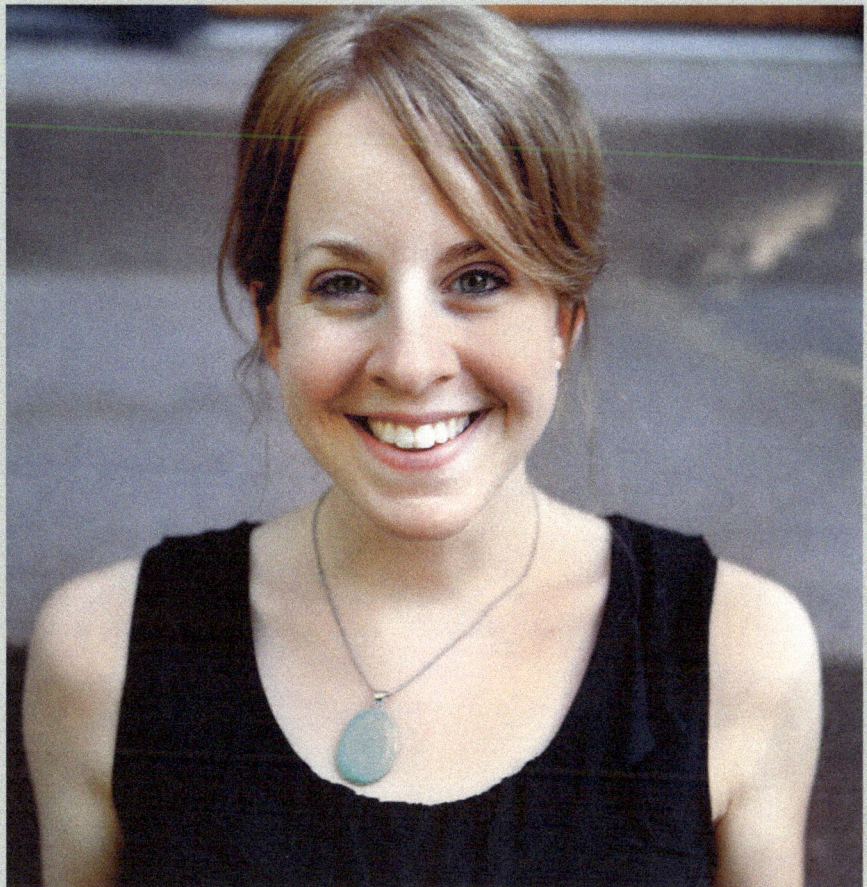

Leah Koenig is an expert when it comes to Jewish cuisine; she lives with her family in New York.

Wat is an Ethiopian dish that is not necessarily Jewish. All Ethiopians eat it, but over the decades Ethiopian Jews have adapted it for Sabbat. Although Leah had eaten Ethiopian food before, she had never connected to it in a personal way. However, the moment she and her friend cooked Doro Wat for Sabbat, with children running around them and the smell of stewing onions filling the kitchen, Leah felt overcome with a strange sense of the familiar. She'd experienced such sites, smells, and sounds before.

That is the most important thing she has learned over the years. The breadth of global Jewish cuisine offers cohesion and a connection with people across many different cultures. As part of that, she's also acquired dishes that aren't from her family, but that she loves nonetheless. Shakshuka, for example, a North African dish that is very popular in Israel and which Leah now

cooks regularly for supper. "Partly it's weird," she observes, "because I realize that I don't own this dish. But as an American, you're used to it. Lasagna is no more mine than tacos. Cook it and enjoy it anyway!"

Leah likes to work with traditional recipes, which she modernizes and spices up with a little love and patience. Like her potato latkes, which she serves with apple-date chutney and cinnamon sour cream. Latkes originate from Eastern Europe, where potato pancakes are often served with apple compote. In German-speaking countries, too, there are countless variations of this dish. In Israel, they are eaten at the Hanukkah Festival of Lights, where they commemorate the eight miraculous days when the oil of the menorah burned. Leah served her latkes with a chutney, which is a bit more modern than the usual apple compote, and the cinnamon adds a special touch to the sour cream that

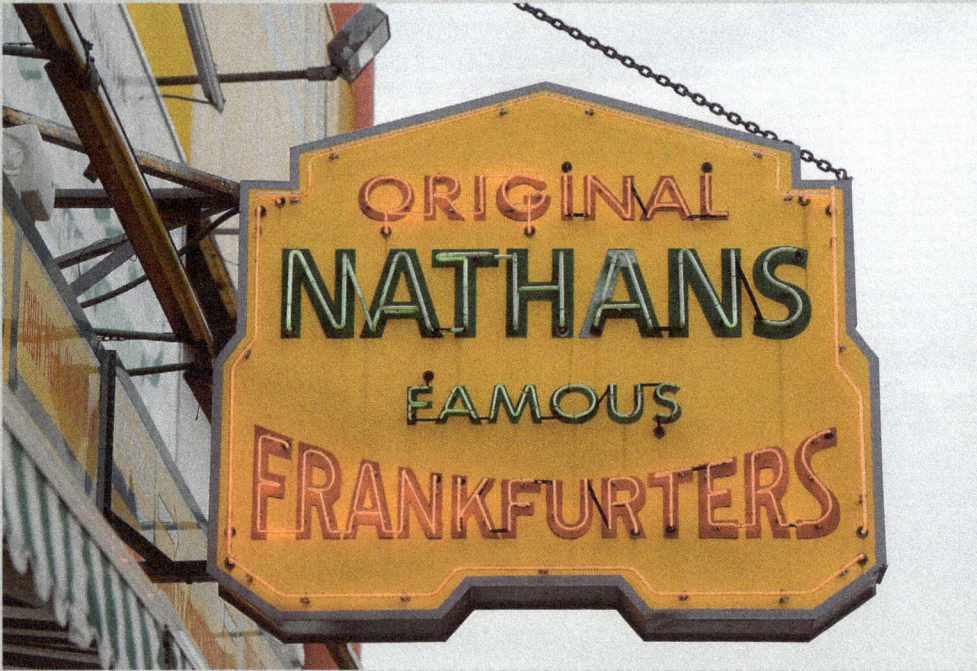

New York City—a city rich in various, global culinary traditions

enhances the entire dish. Another dish you'll often find in Leah's kitchen is classic Jewish mandel bread. Only she uses walnuts in the dough instead of almonds. The pastry is easy to prepare and can be stored for a long time, so you always have something on hand in case unexpected guests drop by for coffee or tea. It also makes a wonderful after-dinner snack, together with a small glass of schnapps.

Ashkenazi food will always be part of Leah and her connections to her ancestors, but today she likes to serve it with the freshness of the Middle East. In her kitchen, the potato kugel often sits next to the roasted red bell pepper salad. The freshness balances the heartiness of Ashkenazi food well. Even in professional kitchens, you can find this mix of Sephardic and Ashkenazic ingredients and recipes.

We live in an increasingly globalized world. Food is just one of many ways to celebrate that. It's important to Leah, however, that we don't allow globalization to break the connection between tradition and food: tradition is part of what gives food its meaning. Maintaining Jewish culinary tradition while adapting it to the modern, globalized world can sometimes be a difficult act to pull off. Jewish cooking has always been subject to adaption; everyone plays with its recipes and changes them a bit. Leah is nonetheless motivated to try. She finds out everything she can about the origins of her recipes and to communicate that as best as she is able in her cooking and in her writing. History, she maintains, is what gives food its meaning.

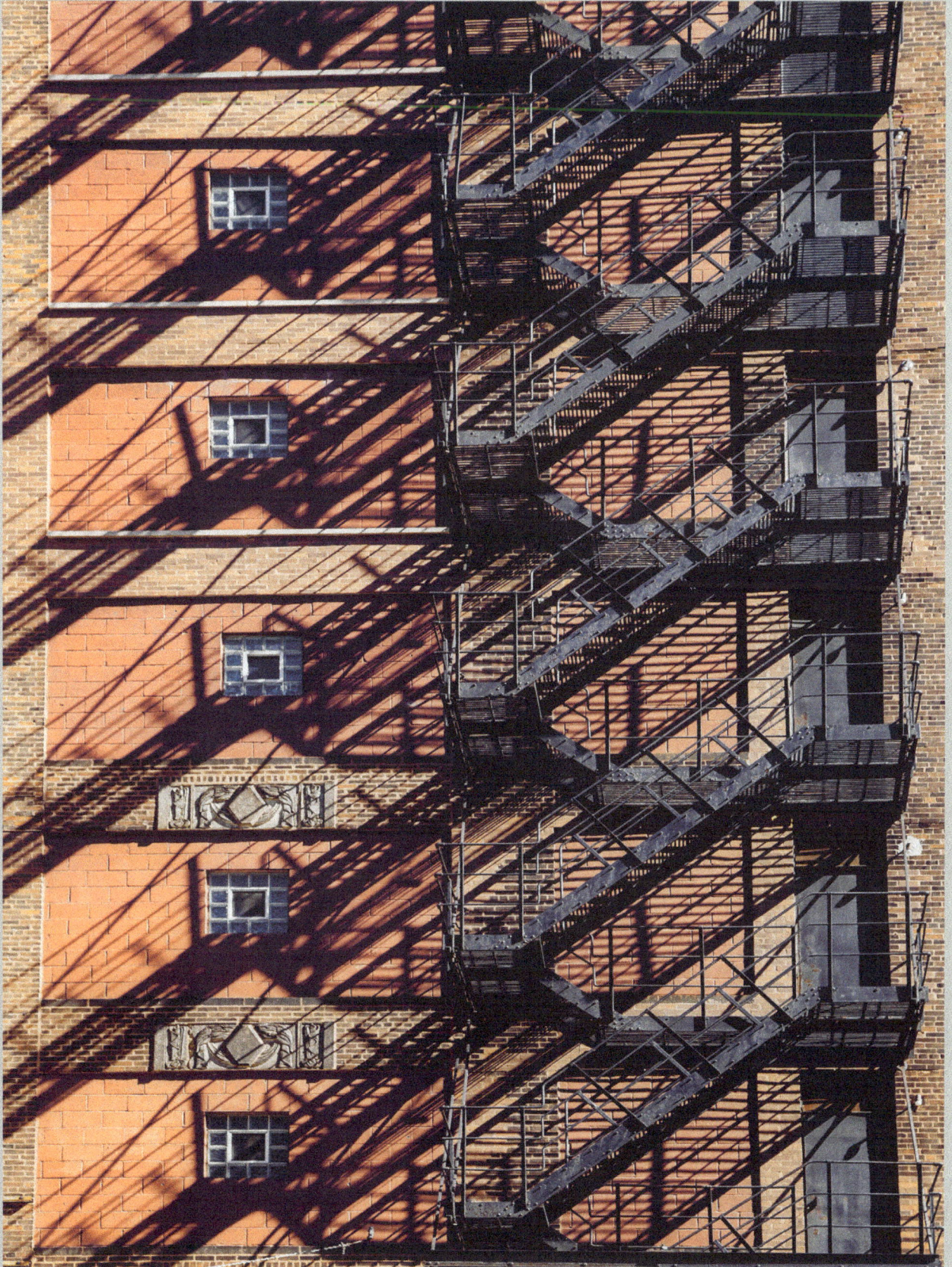

LATKES
— POTATO PANCAKES WITH APPLE-DATE CHUTNEY

FOR 4 PERSONS
PREPARATION: 45 MIN.

CHUTNEY
2 sweet but tart apples, such as Honeycrisp or Pink Lady
1 small onion
¼ cup (60 g) dried dates, pits removed
1 large piece of fresh ginger, 2 inches
¼ cup (60 mL) white wine vinegar
½ cup (100 g) brown sugar
2 tablespoons liquid honey
½ teaspoon ground allspice
Grated zest of 1 organic lemon

POTATO PANCAKES
¾ lb (400 g) potatoes
1 medium onion
Salt
1/3 cup (45 g) pastry flour
2 eggs
Freshly ground black pepper
4-5 tablespoons vegetable oil

CINNAMON CREAM
½ cup (120 g) sour cream
½ teaspoon ground cinnamon
1 teaspoon maple syrup

CHUTNEY

Peel, quarter, and core the apples and cut into small chunks. Dice the onion. Finely chop the dates. Peel the ginger and finely grate. Put everything in a medium saucepan. Add the white wine vinegar, brown sugar, honey, allspice, and 1 teaspoon of freshly grated lemon zest. Cover the pot with a lid and simmer the chutney at a low temperature for 10-15 minutes, until the apple is soft and the chutney has a thick consistency. If necessary, allow chutney to cook longer without a lid if mixture has not thickened. Keep the apple-date chutney lukewarm.

POTATO PANCAKE

Peel and coarsely grate the potatoes and the onion. Place in a medium bowl, lightly salt and let sit for 10 minutes, then firmly squeeze the mixture with your hands to drain all excess water. Then squeeze the mixture vigorously with your hands and drain off the water. Add the flour and the eggs, mix thoroughly and season with salt and freshly ground pepper. Heat the vegetable oil in a skillet over medium heat. Pour in 1 heaping tablespoon of potato mixture at a time and flatten into a pancake about 4 inches in diameter. Cook the potato pancakes in batches until golden brown on both sides.

CINNAMON CREAM

Stir together the sour cream, cinnamon, and maple syrup.

TO SERVE

Arrange the latkes on a large platter. Top with a few dollops of the cinnamon cream and the lukewarm apple-date chutney and serve hot.

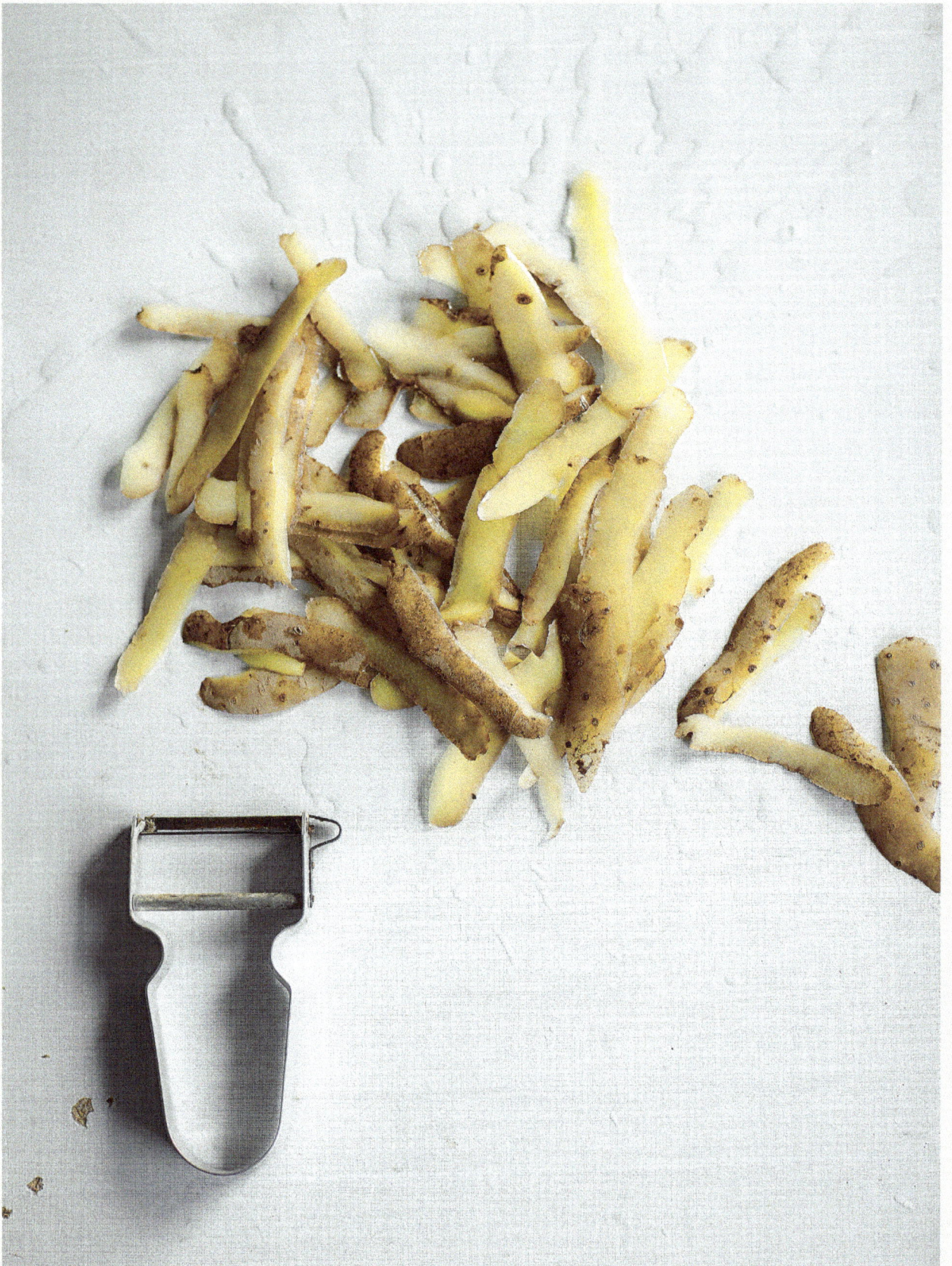

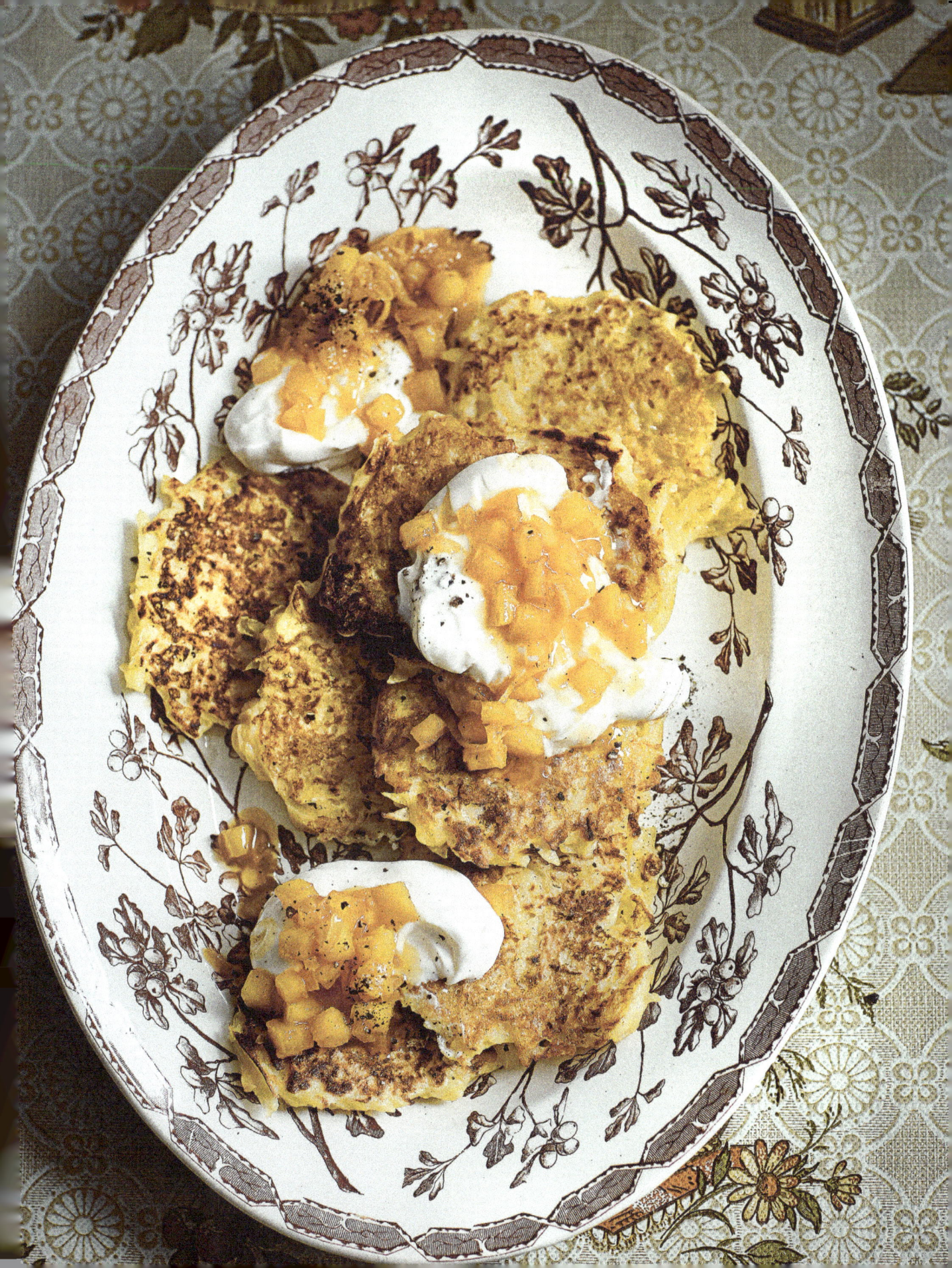

WALNUT MANDEL BREAD

MAKES ABOUT 40 PIECES
PREPARATION: 20 MIN.
BAKING TIME: 30 MIN.

DOUGH

1 ½ cups (180 g) all-purpose
    flour
½ teaspoon baking powder
½ teaspoon baking soda
¼ teaspoon salt
½ cup (110 g) butter, softened
½ cup (100 g) sugar
2 eggs
½ teaspoon vanilla extract
½ teaspoon lemon juice
½ cup (50 g) walnuts, finely
    chopped
Flour for work surface

FINAL STEPS

1/3 cup (65 g) sugar
1 tablespoon ground
    cinnamon
Powdered sugar

DOUGH

1. Preheat the oven to 350°F and line a baking sheet with parchment paper.
2. Sift the flour, baking powder, baking soda, and salt in a medium bowl. Put the softened butter and sugar in a separate mixing bowl and beat for 2 minutes until fluffy. Gradually add the eggs, vanilla extract, and lemon juice, and continue beating. Stir in the flour mixture in two stages until a somewhat sticky dough is formed. Finally, stir in the walnuts.
3. Divide the dough into 2 portions and form each into a long, flat log (9 x 4 inches and ½-inch thick) between 2 layers of lightly floured plastic wrap. Place the two logs onto the lined baking sheet and remove the plastic wrap. Bake for about 20 minutes and bread is lightly browned on top. Remove from the oven and allow to cool for 5 minutes, then cut into slices about ½-inch thick.

FINAL STEPS

Mix the sugar and the cinnamon in a small bowl. Place the slices of bread on the baking sheet with the cut sides down and sprinkle with the cinnamon sugar. Then return to the oven and bake for another 10 minutes. Let the bread slices cool and sprinkle with a little powdered sugar before serving.

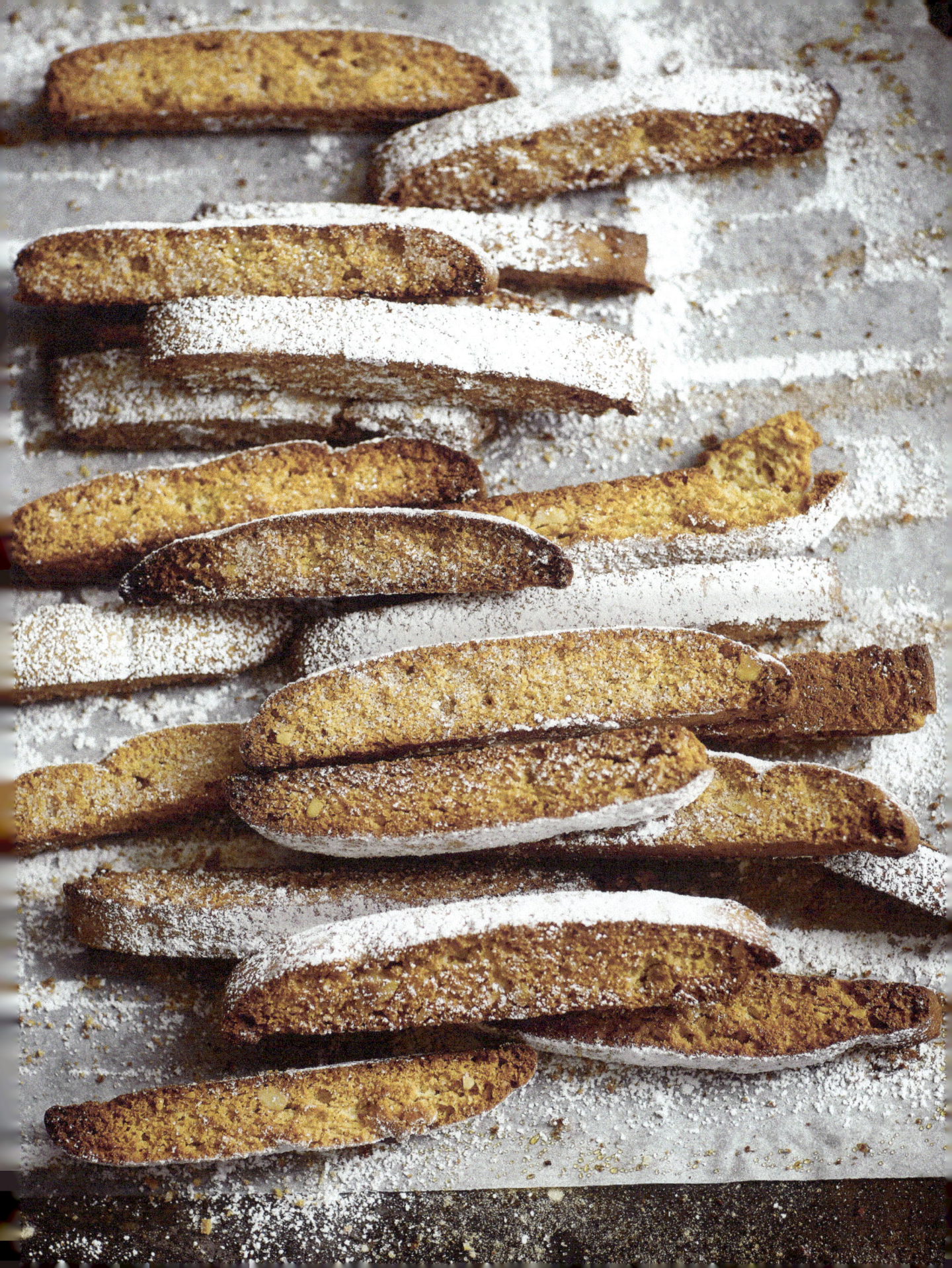

ANNE KORNBLUT,
San Francisco

RECIPES AS TALMUD

Anne Kornblut is Vice President of Global Curation at Facebook since 2015. Before that she worked for twenty years as an editor, book author, and Pulitzer-prize winning journalist at the Washington Post, the Boston Globe, and the New York Times. Her work may be demanding, but she always finds time for cooking and sharing her love for food and her Jewish heritage.

Food didn't always play a big part in her life, though. In her upbringing in the suburbs of Virginia just outside Washington D.C., food was linked mostly with special occasions, like the brisket her grandmother prepared whenever they visited, or the traditional food served at the holidays. As she puts it, she didn't grow up with a real "kitchen culture." That came later, when she and her sister began to explore their Jewish roots partly through food and discovered love for cooking.

In her own home, however, food is a central conduit for passing on her heritage and bringing the family together. Her two children, nine and ten years old, already know their way around the kitchen, and the basics of cooking, especially Jewish dishes. Anne has made a point of passing this knowledge onto her children. Her passion for cooking extends beyond the bounds of her own family, to include her colleagues at work. At Facebook she founded a popular cookbook club.

On the weekends, Anne loves to prepare her BBQ brisket. The dish requires that you get your hands on the boned side of the brisket, something best ordered from a trusted butcher. Although she doesn't smoke it, the way they do in many restaurants, she compensates for that by integrating a smoky BBQ sauce. To reach its juicy, savory best, brisket needs to cook for several hours. But the anticipation is part of the pleasure. You put it on in the morning and then enjoy it in the evening. Served with a salad and some roasted potatoes, it makes for a special weekend meal to enjoy with your family.

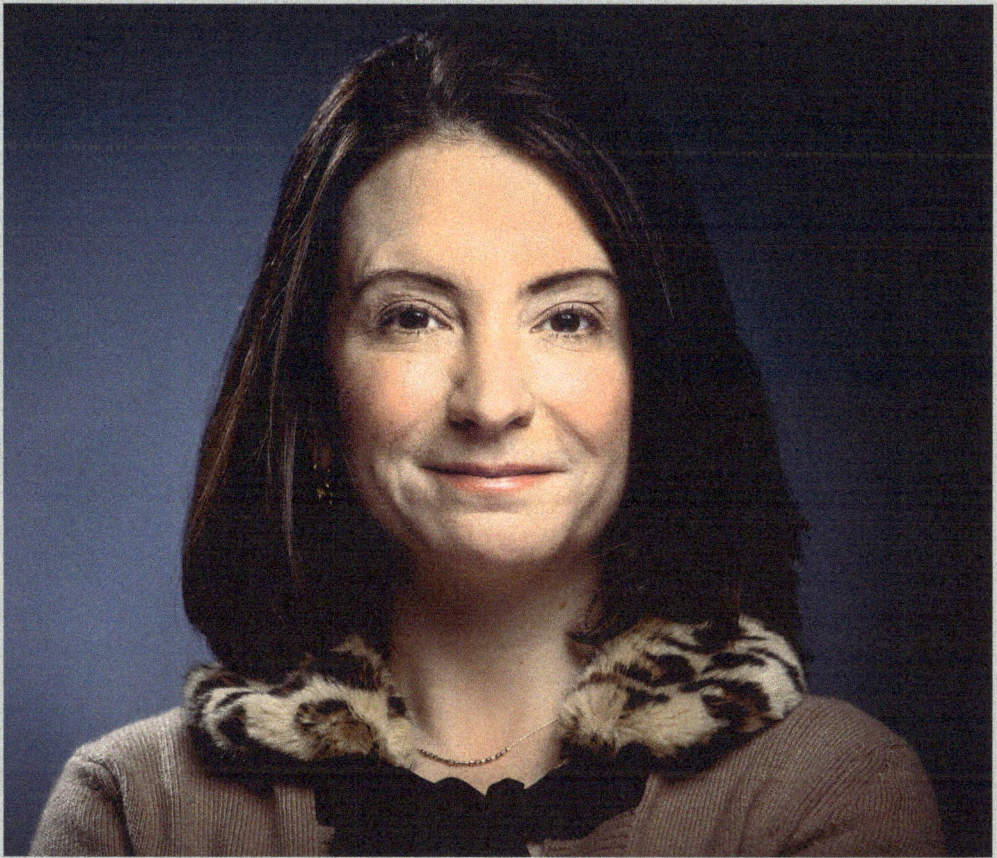

Anne Kornblut is a passionate home chef. She takes pleasure in preparing dishes inspired by her Jewish heritage.

Anne has many vivid memories of certain Jewish foods from her childhood. To take but one example, she will forever link gefilte fish with her father. "Gefilte fish helped me understand how different foods can evoke different emotions and memories. Even though my father has been dead for over 25 years, to this day I can't eat gefilte fish without thinking of him. He loved gefilte fish so much because it reminded him of his own parents."

More recently, Anne inherited a treasure trove of recipes from her husband's mother, Betty Cohen, and grandmother, Jean Cohen. "All of her recipes were carefully documented; they are the Talmud of our family: often studied and discussed." Betty had one ironclad rule: the kugel must not contain raisins! Betty also had an incredible number of kitchen tricks up her sleeve. Sometimes it meant adding a little more butter to a dish, sometimes a whole extra egg. Betty also knew how to make any dish appealing and to make the most of anything on hand. "From a handful of figs and a goat cheese spread, she would whip up an appetizer that was as wonderful as you'd find in any restaurant." Anne picked up Betty's habit of cleaning out the refrigerator by declaring everything "on sale" and mixing it into a sort of mélange. That way, not a bite went to waste.

Food is like language or music, observes Anne. "We pass onto our children the knowledge and act of cooking, whether we mean to or not. It's almost by accident. That makes it one of the more authentic gestures that we share with other people. And it's a knowledge that is shared across generations. I like to imagine how my ancestors ate similarly to how we do today. It makes me happy to know that we have that in common. Like a prayer or a song."

BBQ-BRISKET

SERVES 4
PREPARATION: 30 MIN.
MARINATING TIME: 1-2 DAYS
COOKING TIME: 8 - 9 HRS.

BRISKET

3 1/2 lb (1.5 kg) brisket (beef brisket)
2 teaspoons garlic powder
Salt
Freshly ground black pepper
1 cup (200 mL) smoky BBQ sauce
2 medium onions
4 garlic cloves
1 tablespoon neutral vegetable oil

TO SERVE

2-3 tablespoons zhug, if desired (see recipe "Zhug" on p. 22)

BRISKET

1. Season the beef brisket with the garlic powder, salt, and freshly ground pepper. Place in a large plastic bag and add the BBQ sauce, then seal the bag tightly, rotating the brisket so that it is evenly coated in the sauce. Place the meat in the refrigerator and marinate for 1-2 days.

2. After 1-2 days, remove brisket from refrigerator and preheat oven to 250°F.

3. Cut the onions into ½-inch thick slices. Peel the garlic cloves. Heat the vegetable oil in a cast iron pot or roasting pan and sauté the onions and whole garlic cloves in it for about 5 minutes until golden brown. Remove meat from the plastic bag and set aside the bag with the marinating sauce. Place the meat on top of the onions in the pot or roasting pan. Add 1 cup water to bag with marinating sauce and gently shake bag to incorporate. Pour over the meat and onions. Cover with a lid and cook for 8-9 hours until the meat is fork tender.

4. Transfer the meat to a platter and season generously with salt and pepper and serve with some zhug, if desired.

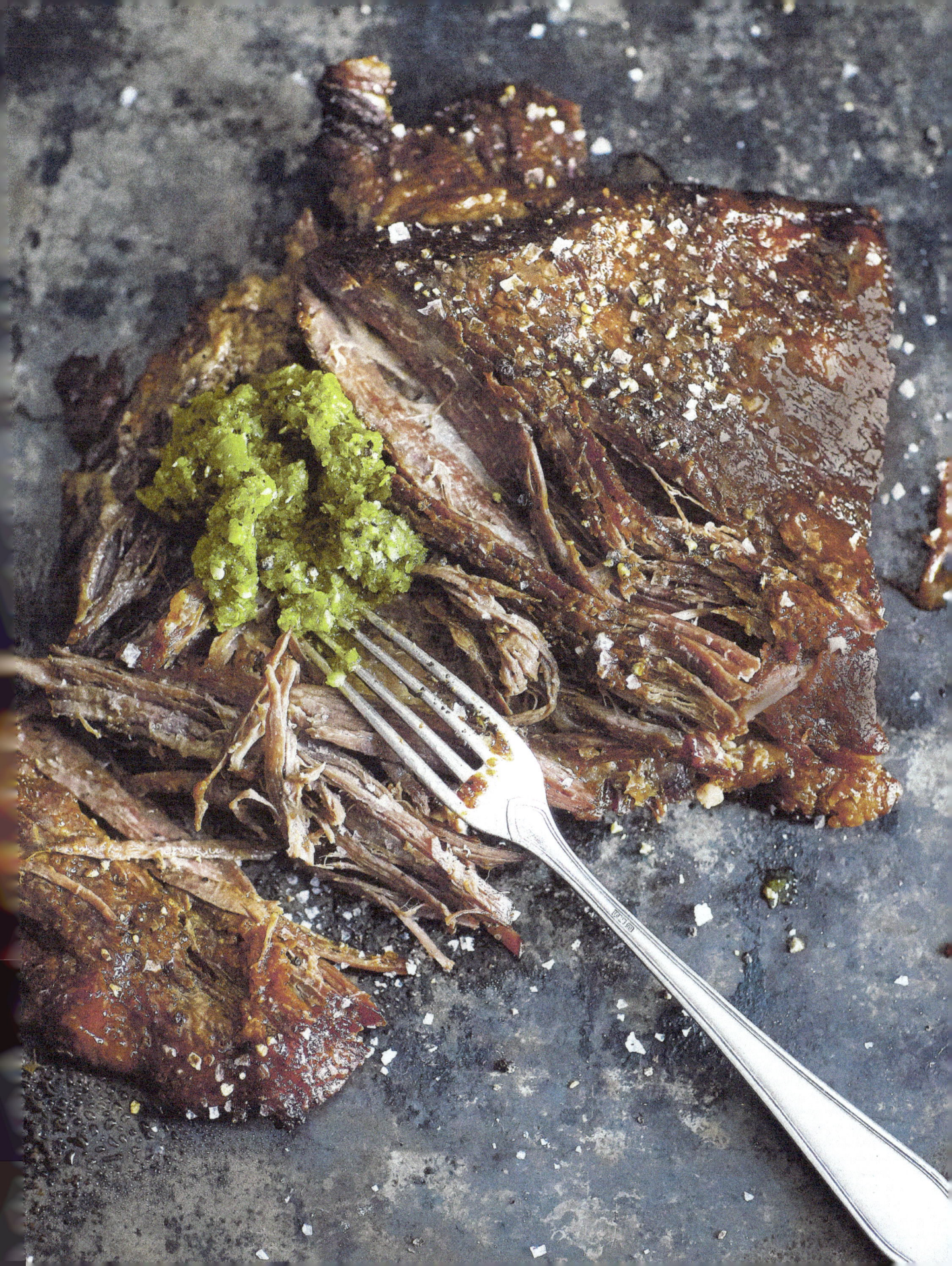

SWEET NOODLE KUGEL

SERVES 6
PREPARATION: 25 MIN.
BAKING TIME: 60 MIN.

SWEET KUGEL

1 tablespoon butter, softened
12 oz (360 g) pasta (such as tagliatelle or fusilli)
6 eggs
1 cup (200 g) cottage cheese
1 2/3 cups (400 mL) milk
1 cup (240 mL) cream
1 cup (200 g) cream cheese
¾ cup (150 g) sugar
1 teaspoon vanilla extract
1 pinch of salt

TOPPING

¼ cup (50 g) sugar
½–1 teaspoons ground cinnamon

SWEET KUGEL

1. Preheat the oven to 350°F. Grease a 9 x 13-inch baking dish with softened butter and set aside.
2. Cook the pasta according to the package instructions so that it still has some bite, al dente.
3. In the meantime, whisk the eggs, cottage cheese, milk, cream, cream cheese, sugar, vanilla extract. and salt in a large bowl until smooth.
4. Drain the pasta, let cool a bit and add to egg mixture in the bowl. Mix everything together well. Pour the pasta mixture into the baking dish and spread evenly.

TOPPING

1. In a small bowl, mix the sugar and cinnamon. Sprinkle evenly over the pasta in the baking dish. Bake for about 1 hour.
2. Remove from oven. Let cool for at least 10 minutes before serving.

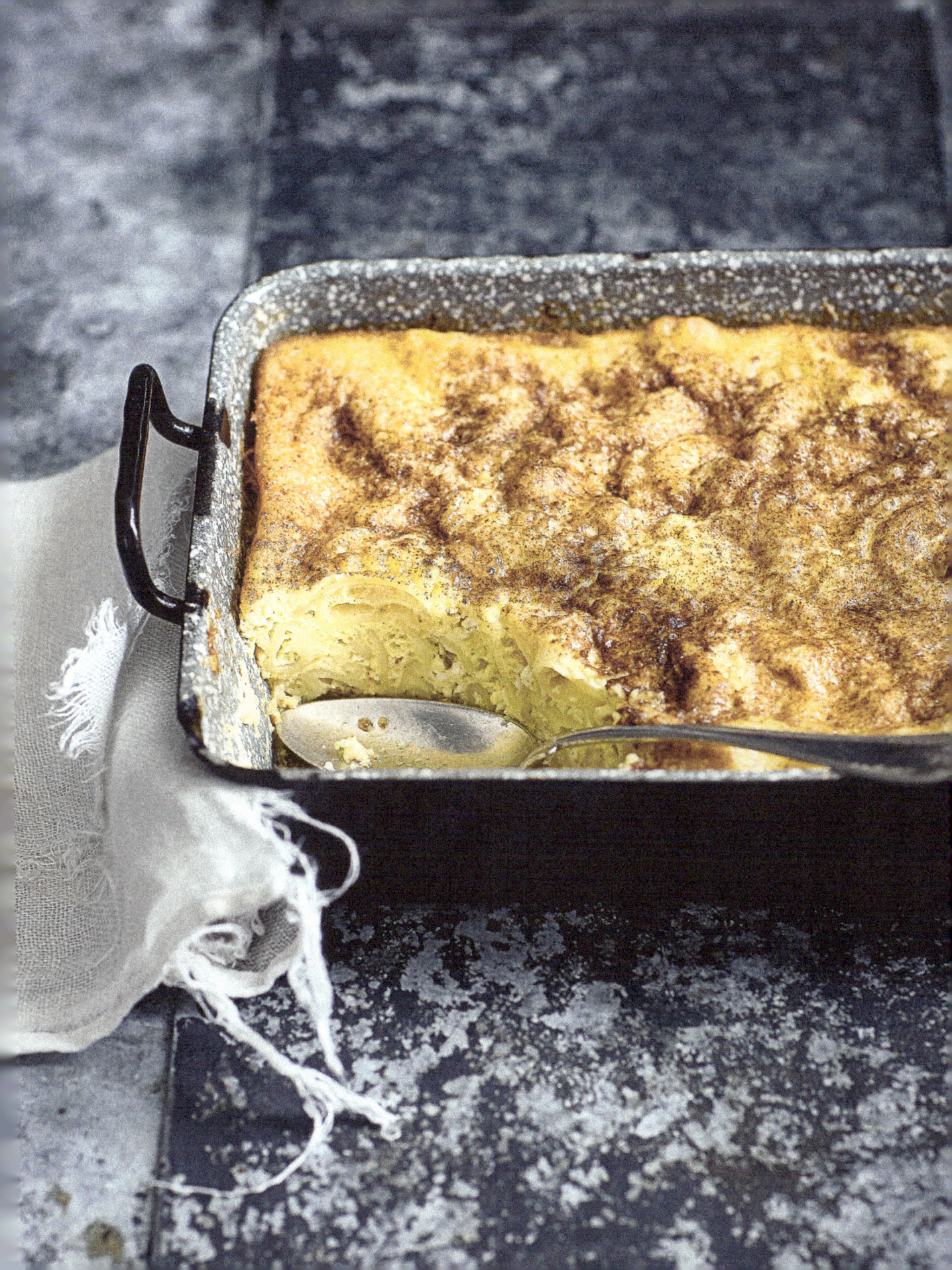

LIZ ALPERN & JEFFREY YOSKOWITZ, New York

JEWISH RECIPES FOR A NEW GENERATION

Liz Alpern and Jeffrey Yoskowitz are icons of Eastern European Jewish cuisine in New York. In 2012 they founded the culinary project, "The Gefilteria" with the aim of making classic Ashkenazi dishes like gefilte fish, which had a reputation as being outdated, bland, and unhealthy, accessible to a whole new generation. As part of their mission to update old-world recipes for the modern world, Jeffrey and Liz cater parties, give workshops, write books, and travel the world.

Liz and Jeffrey met in 2010 at a mutual friend's Sabbat dinner in New York. Jeffrey was a freelance writer who also imported gourmet goods from Israel. Liz was about to move to Washington D.C. to work on various projects related to food. They quickly realized that they shared a love of Ashkenazi food; they were the only ones in their circle of friends who had even the slightest interest in the topic. They both lamented the fact that people dismissed as bad for you the dishes that they had grown up with and loved. Hardly anyone appreciated or cooked Ashkenazi anymore.

They attended a Jewish food conference together, where one of the themes was how traditional Jewish food might be reconciled with a modern lifestyle. In their discussions during the conference and afterwards, they talked a lot about how when it came cooking for the Jewish holidays, people abandoned the values they held dear in daily life. To take but one example, no one paid attention to whether the fish used to prepare gefilte fish had been sustainably harvested. But details like that are important to consider. That's when they started cooking together. They began with gefilte fish. They wanted fish that had been sustainably caught, was fresh, and modern in its presentation. They experimented for a year. What started as gefilte fish soon became other dishes. Drawing on the same principles, they made borscht, pickled and fermented vegetables, and beverages. They also

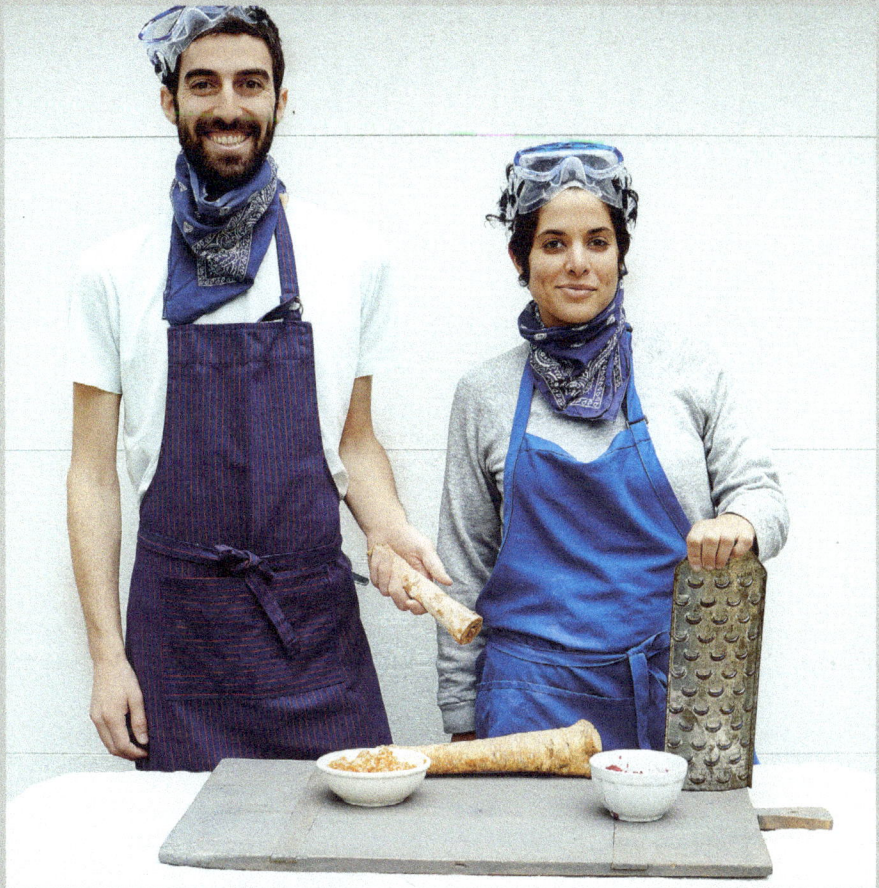

New York natives Liz Alpern and Jeffrey Yoskowitz are reimagining Eastern European Jewish cuisine and giving classic dishes a modern twist

undertook extensive research on the origins of Jewish cuisine and the history of modern cooking. "We thought we needed to adapt Jewish recipes to reflect our modern attitude toward food. Yet this was already ingrained in the cuisine," they note. Some of it was simply lost due to American industrialization. That's when they decided to embark on a mission to share their updated classics and knowledge through the venture, The Gefilteria.

They were excited not only to update classics for those who were already familiar with them but to introduce dishes like gefilte fish and blintzes to people who had perhaps never even heard of them. They traveled to sell their products at various street markets, opened pop-up restaurants, and led workshops. They also co-wrote a cookbook, The *Gefilte Manifesto: New Recipes for Old World Jewish Foods*—a natural extension of their culinary proselyting. The Gefilteria and the cookbook found a ready audience. The project

received glowing write ups in The New Yorker and The New York Times and USA Today and Newsday singled out The Gefilte Manifesto as one of the "best cookbooks of the year."

Liz and Jeffrey accept that not everyone will be open to their modern take on Jewish classics. They won't let that stop them from introducing people to their products, and more importantly, to their recipes. Many people still don't consider Ashkenazi cuisine as a "cuisine" on equal footing with other global cuisines. "Our goal is to validate our culture. After all, it's a food culture rich in tradition, seasonal, and healthy. Jewish cuisine is not just heavy cholent. We can't reach everyone with our aspirations, and that's okay. But we can reach a lot more people and, most important of all, we can change a lot more minds."

CRISPY CHICKEN WITH TSIMMES

SERVES 3
PREPARATION: 30 MIN.
COOKING TIME: 30-40 MIN.

CHICKEN WITH TSIMMES

2 lb (1 kg) chicken pieces, with
    bones and skin
3 tablespoons freshly grated
    ginger
3 tablespoons liquid honey
2 tablespoons vegetable oil
Salt
Chili flakes
Freshly grated zest of 1 organic
    lemon
1 ½ cups (250 g) prunes, pits
    removed
10 medium (500 g) carrots
1 medium onion
Freshly ground black pepper

TO SERVE

4 sprigs of flat-leaf parsley,
    freshly chopped
Cooked rice or kasha

CHICKEN WITH TSIMMES

1. Preheat the oven to 400°F.

2. Rinse the chicken under running water and pat dry. In a bowl, combine the ginger, honey, 1 tablespoon vegetable oil, 1 pinch salt, 1 pinch chili flakes, and 1 tablespoon freshly grated lemon zest.

3. Heat the remaining vegetable oil (1 tablespoon) in a skillet and cook the chicken pieces on all sides for about 7-8 minutes until golden brown, add salt and place cooked chicken into the bowl with the marinade. Coat the chicken pieces all over with the marinade and set aside. Save the skillet with the oil.

4. Coarsely chop the prunes. Peel the carrots and cut into bite-sized pieces. Cut the onion into thin strips. Reheat the pan with the oil, add the onion and sweat for about 5 minutes on medium-high heat until translucent.

5. Add the carrots and prunes and cook for another 5 minutes. Season everything with salt, freshly ground pepper, and 1 pinch of chili flakes.

6. Place the vegetables in an ovenproof dish. Deglaze the juices in the pan with ½ cup of water, bring to a boil, and pour over the vegetables. Place the marinated chicken on top of the vegetables, skin side up, and bake for 30-40 minutes until crispy and cooked through.

TO SERVE

Sprinkle the finished chicken with fresh chopped parsley and serve with either kasha or rice.

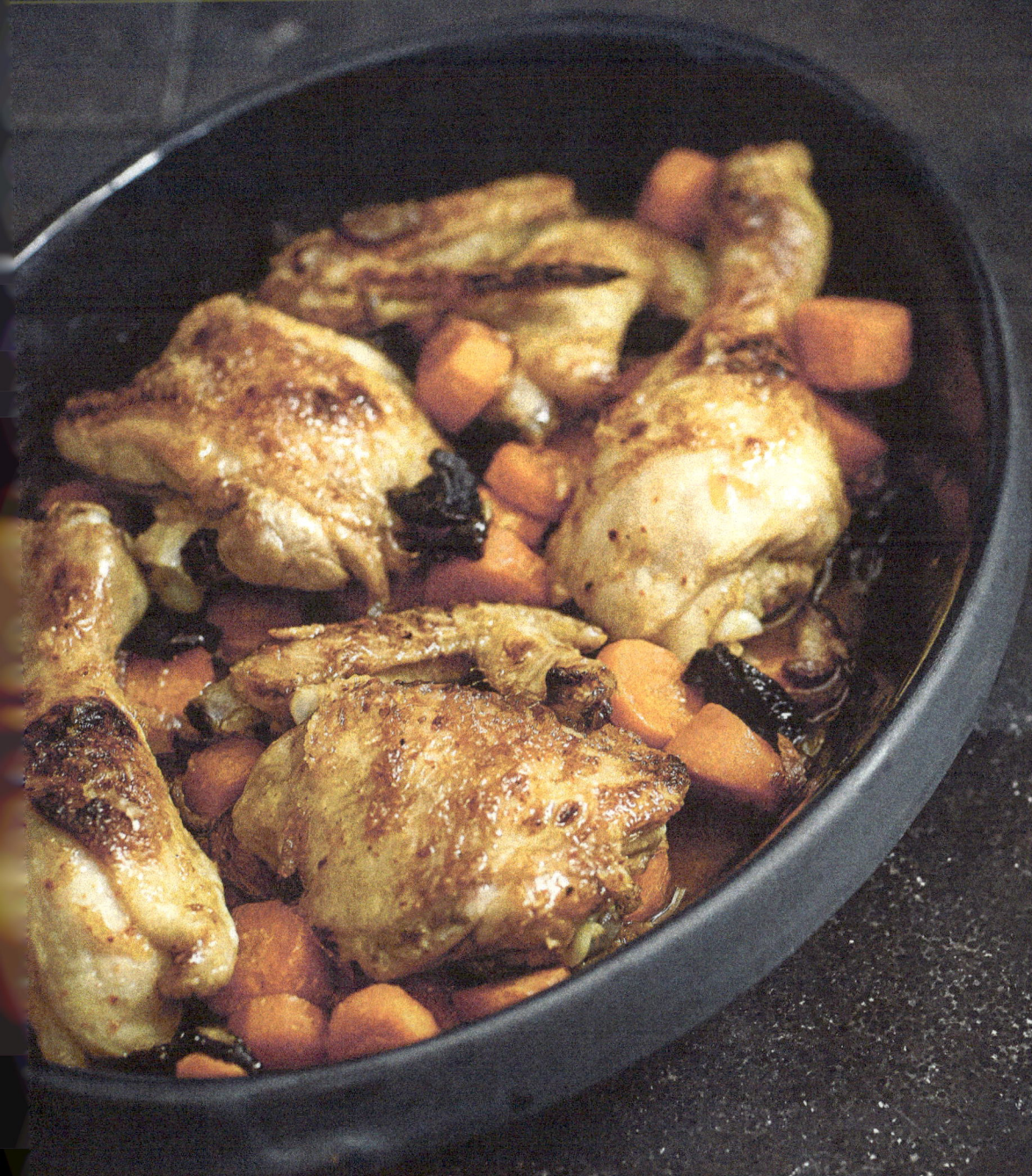

LEKACH
—SPICY HONEY CAKE

MAKES 1 LOAF
(8 ½ x 4 ½ x 2 ½ inches)

PREPARATION: 25 MIN.
BAKING TIME: 60-75 MIN.

CAKE

1 tablespoon butter,
  softened
1 organic orange
1 ½ cups (330 mL) neutral
  vegetable oil (such as
  sunflower oil)
3 eggs
1 1/8 cup (225 g) sugar
¾ cup (225 g) honey
¾ cup (180 mL) coffee,
  lukewarm
1 ½ cup (180 g) pastry flour
1 cup (120 g) rye flour
2 teaspoons baking powder
½ teaspoon baking soda
2 teaspoons ground
  cinnamon
¼ teaspoon ground ginger
¼ teaspoon ground cloves
½ teaspoon salt

GLAZE

1 organic orange
3-4 tablespoons powdered
  sugar

CAKE

1. Preheat the oven to 350°F. Grease the loaf pan with softened butter and lightly dust with flour.
2. Wash the orange and finely zest the peel into a small bowl.
3. In a bowl, whisk together the vegetable oil, eggs, sugar, honey, coffee, and orange zest until smooth. In a separate large bowl, combine the pastry flour, rye flour, baking powder, baking soda, spices, and salt. Make a well in the flour mixture, pour in the egg mixture and mix everything together until a homogeneous batter is formed.
4. Pour the batter into the prepared pan and bake for 60-75 minutes until a fork or toothpick inserted in the center comes out clean, i.e., without any batter clinging to it. If during baking it begins to brown too much, loosely cover it with a layer of aluminum foil.
5. Remove from the oven, place on a rack, and allow to cool in the pan for at least 30 minutes. Once cooled, remove from pan.

GLAZE

Wash the orange and using a grater or peeler, remove long, thin pieces from the rind. In a medium bowl, mix the powdered sugar with a few tablespoons of orange juice until smooth. Pour the orange glaze over the cake and spread. Garnish with the orange zest if desired.

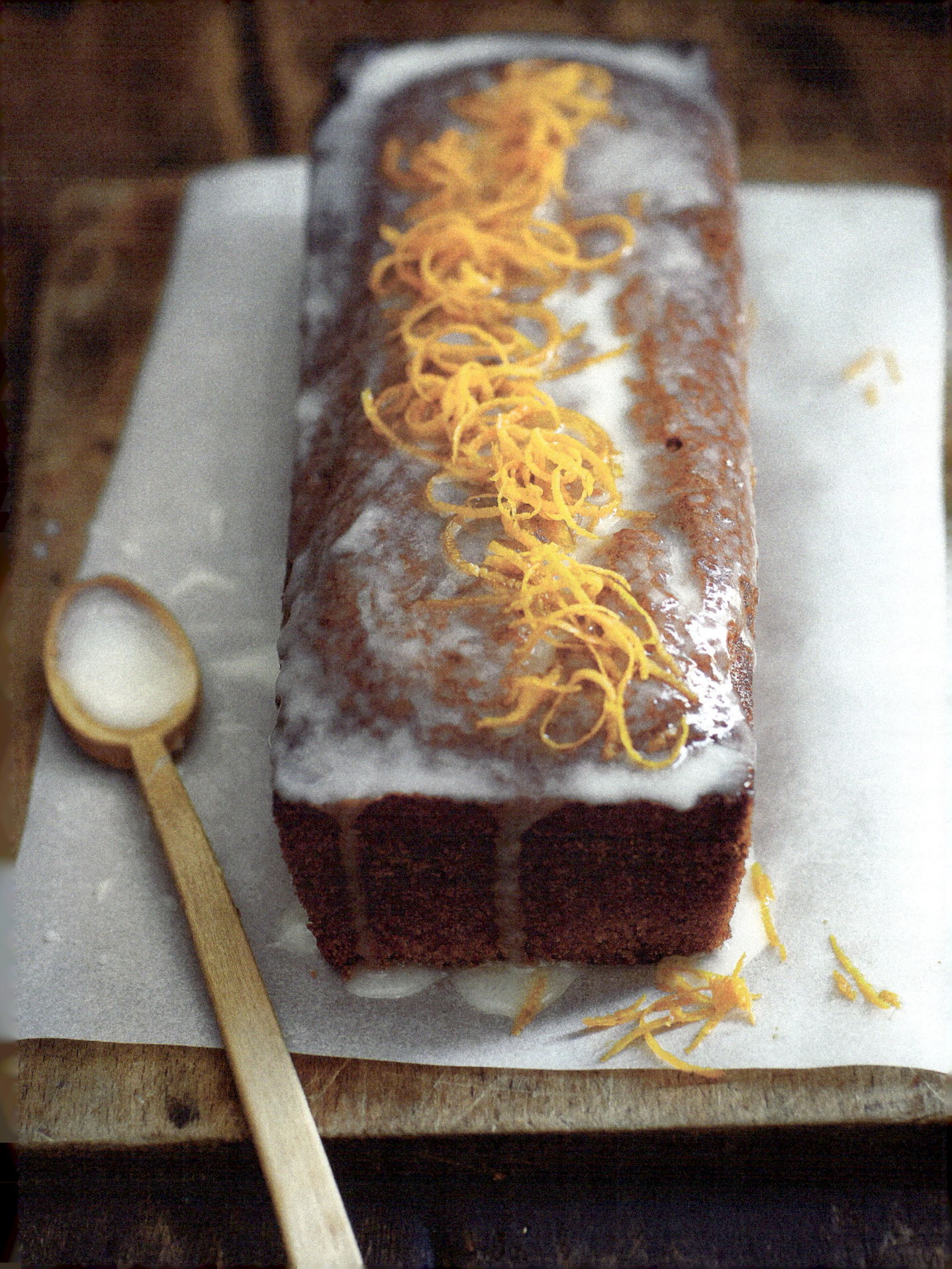

PICKLED HERRINGS

SERVES 4-6
PREPARATION: 10 MIN.
INFUSION: 2 DAYS
DRAINING: 1-3 HRS.

PICKLED HERRINGS
6 fresh herrings, gutted
  and heads removed
1 cup (250 g) salt

PICKLED HERRINGS

1. Wash the herrings thoroughly and pat dry. Sprinkle the bottom of a rectangular mold or baking pan with salt. Place the herrings side by side in the mold or pan and cover with the remaining salt. Then cover with plastic wrap, place a board on top, and weigh it down with something heavy (e.g., butter packets, milk cartons or similar). Place in the refrigerator and let the herrings pickle for 2 days.
2. Before use, remove the herrings from the bed of salt and set in bowl with plenty of cold water. Leave them to soak and desalt for 1-3 hours, then pat dry.

Tip: The preserved herrings are good for frying and for making dishes like fish & chips. They also taste good fried with beans and served with potato salad. In Poland, herrings are preserved with onions, vinegar, pepper, cloves, sugar, and bay leaves for 2 days and served cold with potatoes or bread.

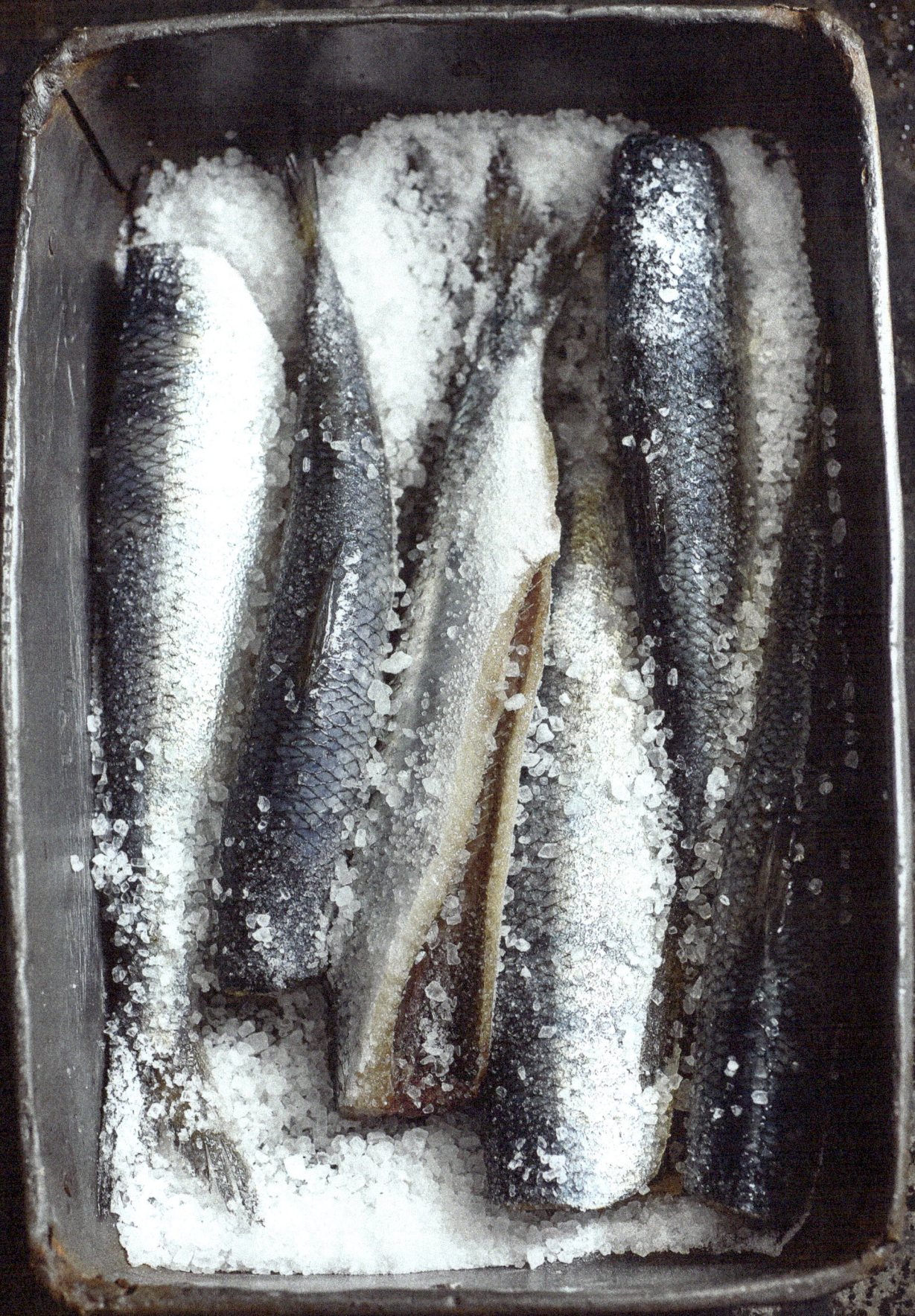

MOLLY YEH, Grand Forks

DISHES WITH A HISTORY

When you live in what feels like the middle of nowhere, you quickly learn to make the dishes you miss the most. At least that's how Molly Yeh felt when she moved from New York City to Grand Forks, North Dakota, to a sugar beet farm in 2014. No more delis, no more restaurants open 24 hours, and no more bagels. Although the blogger has always loved to cook, she blossomed in her farm kitchen and taught herself how to make an impressive number of new dishes. Living in such a rural setting also made her feel more connected to her Jewish roots.

Molly grew up in Chicago and studied in New York. She never felt the need to search for Jewish traditions or food; they were simply part of her life. As a picky child, she refused to eat just about anything green, preferring comfort foods like matzo balls and challah.

When she moved to Grand Forks with her husband, she suddenly had no access to her favorite foods. If she wanted bagels or challah, she had to make them herself. As Molly combed through various recipes, she also did a lot of research, learning about the traditions behind many of her favorite dishes. She discovered such things as the reason why all challah recipes make two loaves and why you braided them. Research and cooking for her non-Jewish husband were both a part of her effort to carry on the traditions of her Jewish roots.

Molly's cooking reflects not only her Jewish but also her Chinese heritage. Her mother is Jewish, and her father is Chinese. In her childhood home and even today, these two very different cuisines have never been separate. Her mother served Chinese dumplings as a side dish alongside latkes and nearly

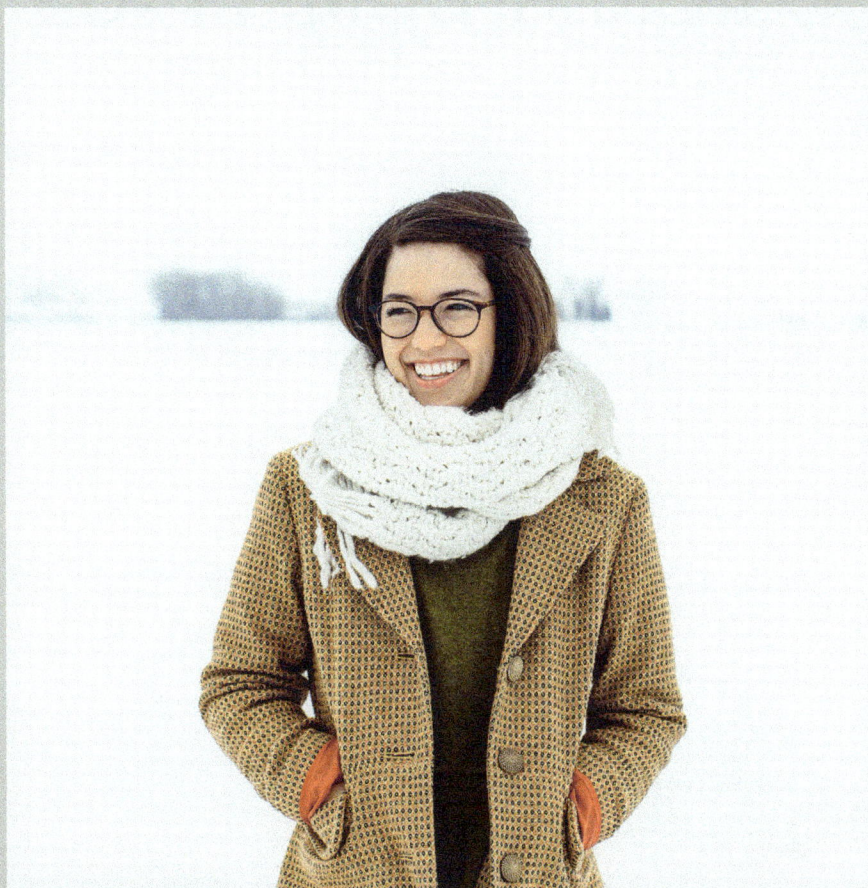

Molly Yeh is an urbanite at heart, but since 2014 she has been living with her American-Norwegian husband on a sugar beet farm in North Dakota.

every dish included soy sauce. Molly inherited her mother's instinctively multicultural and experimental approach. The result is cooking that is original, bright, and colorful. She often combines different flavors just because they taste good together, not because she is trying to stay true to a particular culinary tradition. She'll fill dumplings with hummus, for instance, trusting that it will somehow work out just fine.

In addition to her upbringing and own experiments in her South Dakota kitchen, over the past few years, Molly has also traveled often to Israel. That's where she discovered Israeli-Sephardic cuisine, whose dishes she now counts as among her favorites.

Molly's halva rugelach is a recipe that illustrates her cooking style at its best. It combines the traditional Ashkenazi Eastern European rugelach pastry with Israeli cuisine. Instead of chocolate filling, Molly uses halva spread. Halva is a common ingredient in many Arab countries. Its base mixture is usually made from oil seeds and sugar or honey. Molly uses honey and tahini to give it a distinctive Israeli flavor. Molly especially enjoys the rugelach fresh out of the oven alongside a hot drink.

The food of the diaspora fascinates and inspires Molly, especially dishes with a story behind them. She is grateful for the world that travel has opened up for her. Through her travels she's acquired new recipes and ingredients and knowledge about the history of the Jewish diaspora—all of which she tries to incorporate into her own joyous cooking.

CHICKEN-DUMPLINGS

SERVES 4 /
   MAKES 24 DUMPLINGS
PREPARATION: 50-60 MIN.

DOUGH
2 cups (240 g) pastry flour,
   plus a little more for the
   work surface
1 teaspoon salt
½ cup (120 mL) boiling water
½ cup (120 mL) cold water

FILLING
1 lb (500 g) ground chicken
1 piece fresh ginger, 1-inch
   long
2 spring onions
1 teaspoon sugar
2 teaspoons soy sauce
2 teaspoons light rice
   vinegar
1/3 cup (80 mL) cold chicken
   stock
Salt
Freshly ground black pepper
   Freshly ground black
   pepper

DOUGH

In a large bowl, mix the flour and salt. Using a wooden spoon, slowly stir in the boiling water, then add the cold water. Mix together, then put onto a lightly floured work surface and knead with your hands to form a slightly sticky dough. Cover the dough with a kitchen towel and let it rest at room temperature for about 20 minutes.

FILLING

Place the ground chicken in a bowl. Peel and finely grate the ginger and add to the bowl. Wash and trim the spring onions, chop into thin rings and add to the meat. Add the sugar, soy sauce, rice vinegar, and chicken stock and mix together. Season with salt and freshly ground pepper.

FINAL STEPS

1. Form 24 small balls from the dough and roll them out into thin circles. Place 1 tablespoon of chicken mixture in the center of each dough circle and gently fold in half, forming a crescent shape. Press the edges of the dough firmly together and bend into a banana shape.

FINAL STEPS
5 tablespoons neutral
   vegetable oil
Salt

TUNKA
2 spring onions
¼ cup (60 mL) soy sauce
2 tablespoons light rice
   vinegar
4 tablespoons roasted
   sesame oil
Freshly ground black
   pepper

2. Bring plenty of salted water to a boil in a large pot and cook the dumplings in batches (6-8 at a time) for about 2 minutes until they rise to the surface. Using a slotted spoon, remove the dumplings from the water and set them on a kitchen towel to let the steam from them evaporate.

3. While the steam evaporates, prepare the sauce. Heat the vegetable oil in a large non-stick skillet over medium-high heat. Fry the dumplings until golden brown on all sides.

TUNKA
Wash and clean the scallions and chop them into very fine rings. In a bowl, mix the spring onion rings with the soy sauce, rice vinegar, and sesame oil. Season with freshly ground pepper.

TO SERVE
Divide the fried dumplings among 4 plates, each accompanied by a small bowl of tunka sauce.

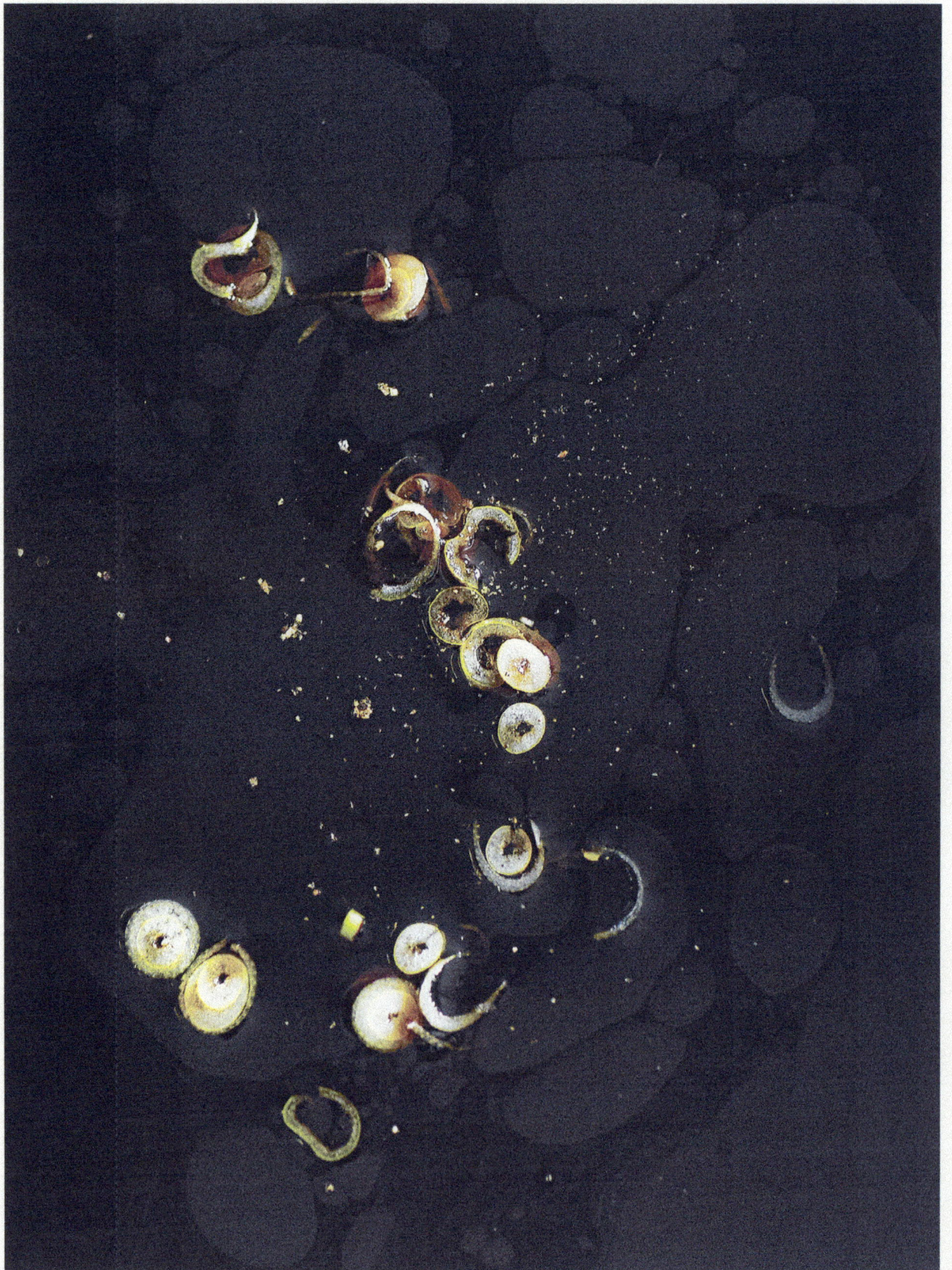

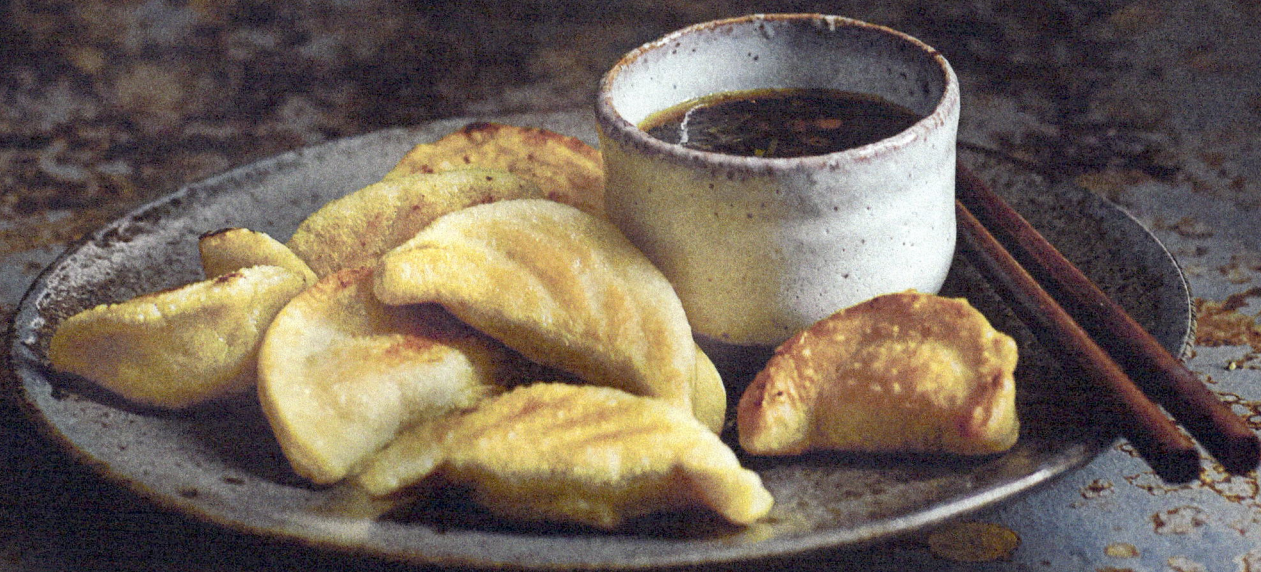

HALVA-RUGELACH

MAKES 24 PIECES
PREPARATION: 50 MIN.
RESTING TIME: 4½ HRS.

DOUGH
14 tablespoons (200 g)
  butter, room temp.
1 1/3 cups (240 g) cream
  cheese
¼ cup (55 g) sugar
2 egg yolks
1 ½ teaspoons vanilla
  extract
1 teaspoon pure almond
  extract
½ teaspoon salt
3 cups (360 g) pastry flour

FILLING
¾ cup (170 g) tahini
3 tablespoons (55 g)
  honey
1 pinch of salt
1 pinch of ground
  cinnamon

FINAL STEPS
1 egg
1 tablespoon honey
Roasted sesame seeds for
  sprinkling

DOUGH

Place the butter and cream cheese in a large bowl and beat with a hand mixer for 5 minutes until fluffy. Gradually add the sugar and egg yolks, as well as the flavoring extracts and salt, continuing to beat steadily. Finally, sift in the flour and knead everything into a fairly sticky dough. Wrap the dough in plastic wrap and let it rest in the refrigerator for 4 hours.

FILLING

Mix the tahini, honey, salt, and cinnamon in a bowl.

FINAL STEPS

1. Divide the dough in half and roll out each between 2 layers of plastic wrap, about ¼-inch thick, in a circular shape. Chill in the refrigerator for 30 minutes.
2. Preheat the oven to 400°F. Line a baking sheet with parchment paper.
3. Remove the dough from the refrigerator. Beginning with the first one, set on a lightly floured surface. Spread with the filling and using either a pizza cutter or knife, cut into 12 pieces, the way you would a pie. Starting with the wider end, roll up the triangles to form small croissants and place on the baking sheet. Repeat with the second pastry circle.
4. For the glaze, whisk the egg, honey, and 1-2 tablespoons of water in a small bowl until smooth. Brush the croissants with the glaze and sprinkle with sesame seeds. Bake for 15-20 minutes until golden brown.

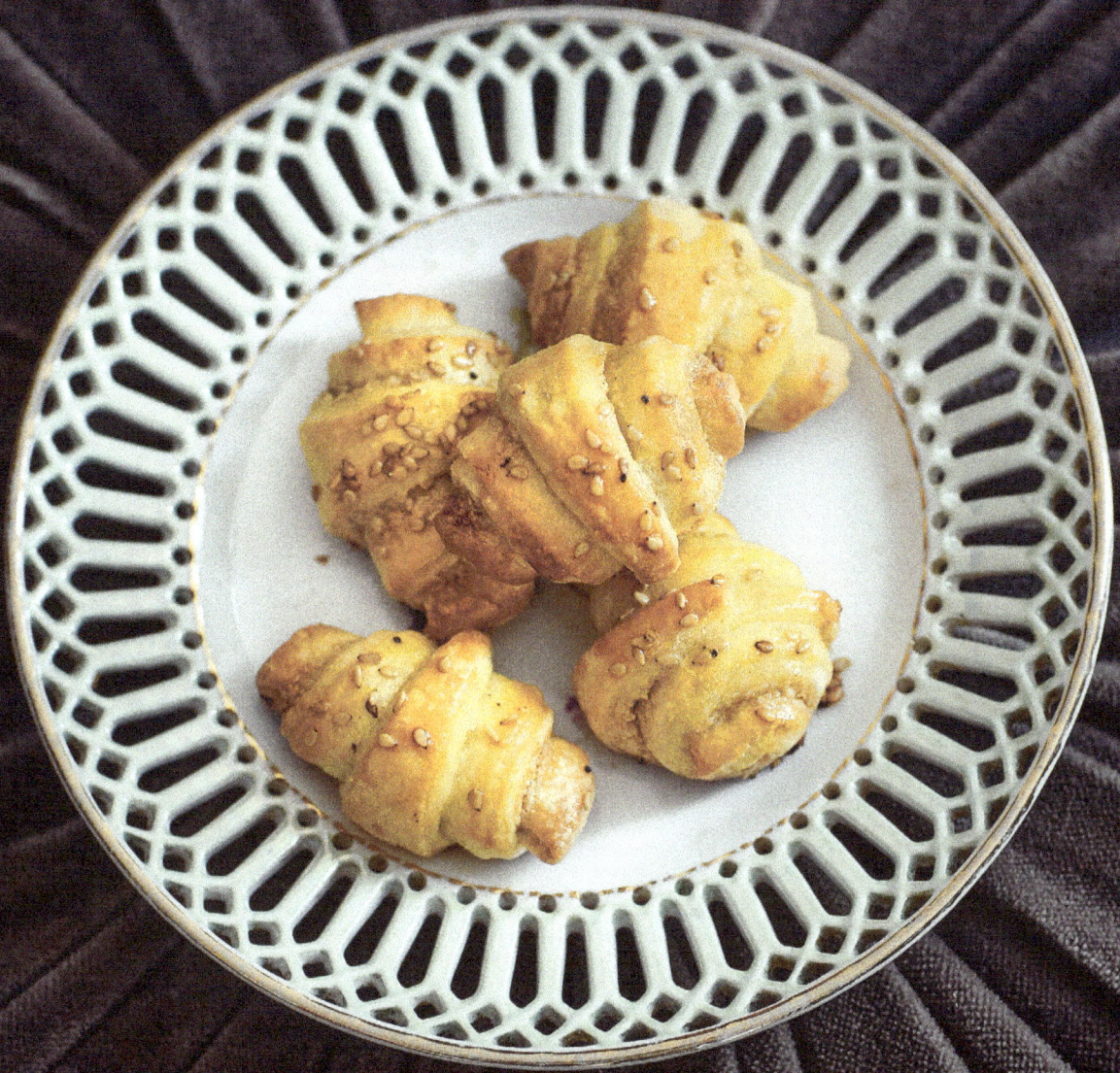

MATZO-BREI PANCAKES

SERVES 2 /
  MAKES 8 PANCAKES
PREPARATION: 25 MIN.

PANCAKES
2 unleavened matzo cra-
  ckers
2 eggs
2 tablespoons sugar
½ teaspoon ground
  cardamom
1 teaspoon baking powder
Some butter for frying

TO SERVE
1 ½ cups (250 g) fresh
  mixed berries (such as
  blueberries, raspberries,
  strawberries)
1/3 cup (80 g) Greek
  yogurt
2 tablespoons maple
  syrup
2 sprigs of fresh mint
Powdered sugar

This recipe is a sweet twist on the otherwise neutral tasting matzos that traditionally are the only bread served during Passover.

PANCAKES

1. In a medium bowl, break the matzo crackers into small pieces and cover with lukewarm water. Soak for 5 minutes then squeeze and drain the water and put back in bowl. Add the eggs, sugar, cardamom, and baking powder and mix to a uniform, thick batter.
2. Heat a non-stick skillet over medium-high heat and brush with a little butter. Add 1-2 tablespoons of matzo batter at a time to the pan, spreading them into a circle about 6-inches in diameter. Cook the pancakes until golden brown on both sides.

TO SERVE

Arrange the pancakes on a platter. Top each with fresh berries and a few dollops of yogurt. Drizzle with maple syrup and garnish with mint leaves. Drizzle everything with maple syrup and garnish with the plucked mint leaves. Finally, sprinkle with a little powdered sugar and serve warm.

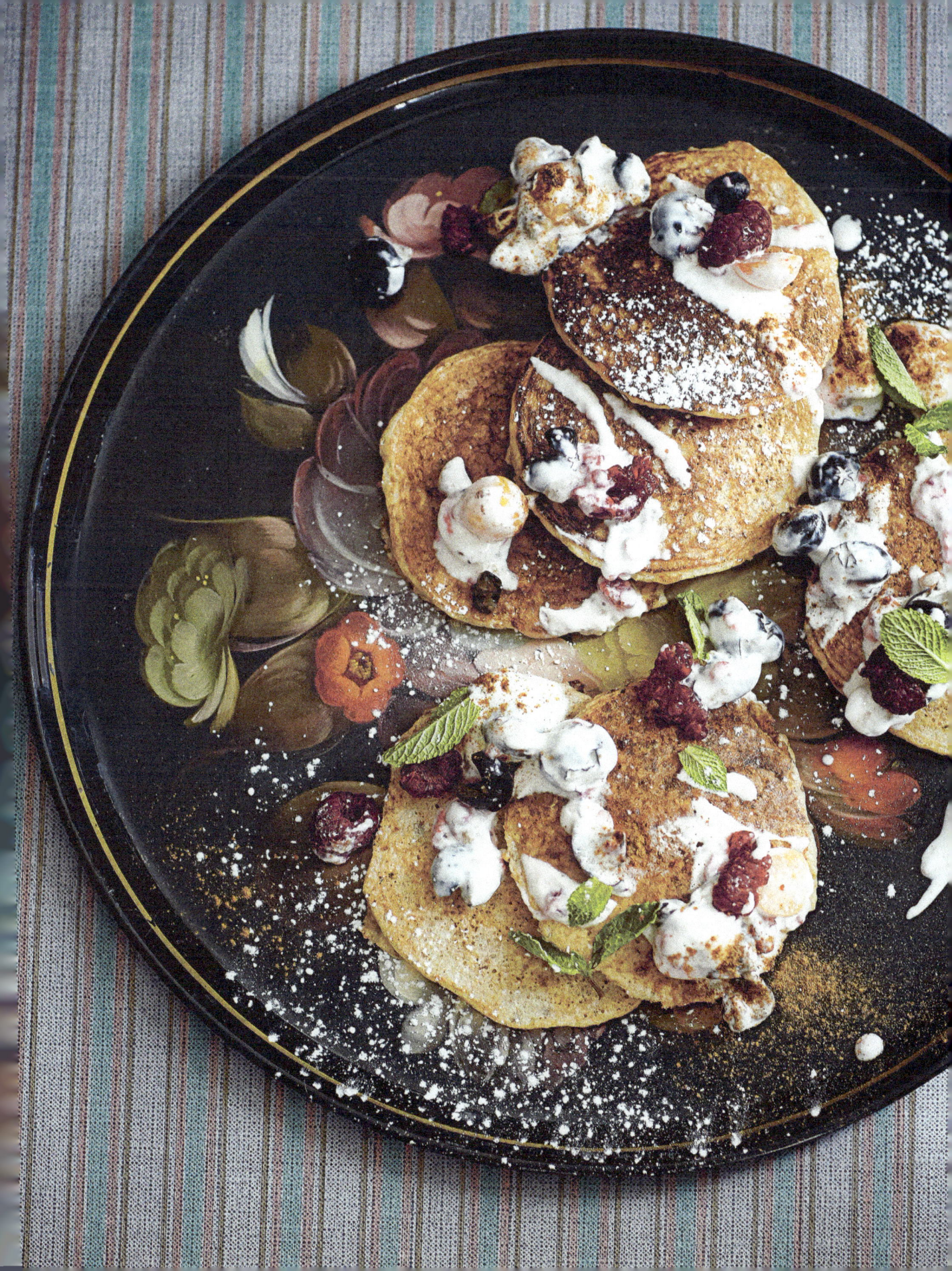

PATRICIA JINICH, Dallas

A JEWISH-MEXICAN-AMERICAN MIX

Barely have you started to ask Patricia Jinich a question before the Jewish-Mexican chef starts telling you about her incredibly interesting family history. The award-winning chef is a well-known television personality, cookbook author, and food journalist. Born in Mexico City, Pati's grandparents immigrated to Mexico from Poland. Everything she knows about Judaism she learned from her grandparents. Her own parents weren't religious; they lived on the fringes of the Jewish community in Mexico City. As a child, she often felt torn between the competing strands of her identity. She felt different, like an outsider. At school she was often teased for being one of the very few blue-eyed children and she also had to deal with a lot of anti-Semitic attitudes and superstitions, which were still common in Mexico back then. People would openly say things like "Jews drink the blood of children and secretly control all of the money in the world." She found it almost a little embarrassing to be Jewish. Her Polish last name also made her stand out from her peers who had Hispanic last names like "Gomez," "Garcia," or "Lopez."

Her grandparents on her mother's side of the family, have an incredibly romantic and unusual history. Her grandfather was born in Bratislava and her grandmother came from Austria. Sometime in the late 1930s, when they were teenagers, they met at a spa town in Central Europe. By chance some mutual friends got together and the two struck up a conversation. The Jewish teenagers joked that they would meet again one day in Mexico if war broke out. When that did eventually happen, her grandfather made his way to Mexico, while everyone else in his family stayed behind, eventually to die in concentration camps.

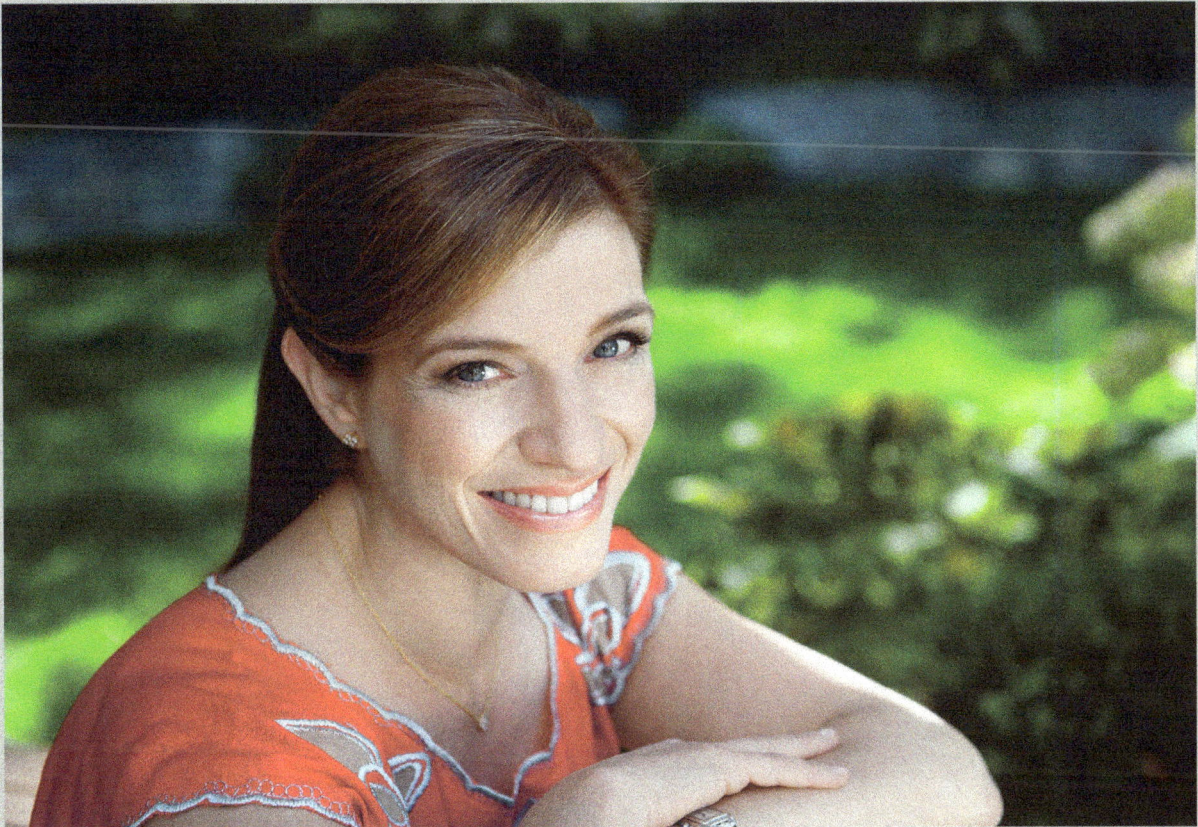

Pati Jinich moved with her family from Mexico to the US and has since brought these three heritages together in her cooking.

Pati's grandmother found her way there too but via a less direct route. When she was 18, and the Nazis had taken power, her family sent her to live with her uncle in Brooklyn. She escaped Nazi Europe just in time, right before her family was transported to a camp. Her grandmother didn't stay in Brooklyn for long; she decided to go to Mexico. Out of sheer desperation, alone, she took a boot to Mexico. She had hardly any money, but by pure chance she met up with Pati's grandfather again in Mexico City, whom she'd only met once in that spa town in Europe. Not long after, they married. Pati's grandmother then began to look for her sister; the only member of her family to survive the camps. Once she had found her, she brought her to Mexico. This great-aunt opened Mexico's first European bakery.

Both of Pati's grandmothers were talented cooks. The Czech-Austrian side of the family were cultivated and made elegant dishes. Her Polish grandparents were somewhat humbler and made more rustic fare. Her Czech-Austrian grandmother often made a duck broth that she served with elegant, small matzo balls. Her Polish grandmother made her matzo-ball soup with a lot of lard and matzo balls that always looked rather lumpy. The matzo-ball soup that Pati makes takes inspiration from her Czech-Austrian grandmother's version. Pati, however, uses jalapeños, something neither her grandmother ever did.

In Mexico City, the Jewish community is very close, and they do and cook a lot together. The Ashkenazi Jews who came to Mexico adapted their cooking to Mexican cooking. They added avocados to egg salad (a sort of Yiddish guacamole); they seasoned matzo-ball soup with jalapeños; and they transformed the plain, beige color of traditional gefilte fish into

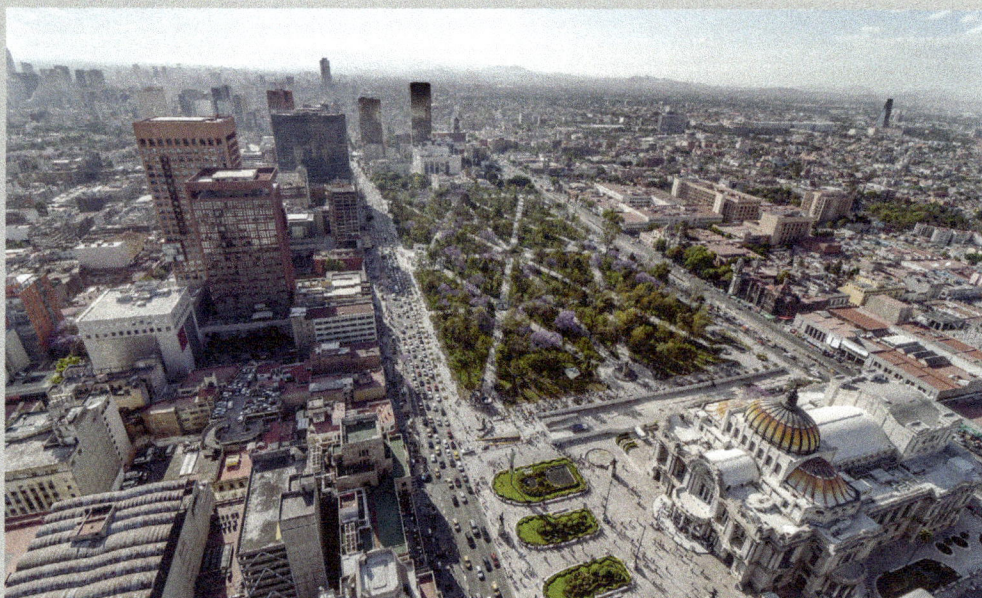

Left: The Dallas skyline
Right: Thanksgiving Square in Dallas

something red, gefilte fish "a la Veracruzana." Pati is especially fond of Mexican gefilte fish, because the dish combines traditional gefilte fish with a red sauce that is popular in Mexico's state of Veracruz. The result is a thick, well-seasoned, tomato sauce, rich in capers, green olives, and mildly pickled chilies.

For a long time, Pati had mixed feelings about Judaism. Although she was proud of her family history, she struggled to make that clear to the outside world. Growing up, she often heard that she didn't look or "act Jewish." Uncomfortable with such accusations, she hid her Jewish origins from new friends. But this ran counter to her strong awareness that her Jewish heritage was an important part of who she was: many members of her family had died for merely being Jewish. Not until much later, when she moved to Dallas with her husband and had children of her own, did she find a way to reconcile

these various, competing parts of her identity. Living in the US raised a whole other set of issues. There she felt like she had to protect her Mexican identity. Now she sees all three of her cultural heritages (Mexican, Jewish, American) as equally strong and equally valuable. It may have taken her a long time to get there, but she now rejoices in the fact that so many heritages "belong to her." Cooking has helped her find a way to blend them together in a harmonious whole.

When it comes to food and culture, she believes that you shouldn't be afraid to look back and appreciate your family history. But you should also keep one eye on the future and incorporate new things: "I like to prepare foods that have meaning for me and my family. Every Friday night I know my sister is probably in Mexico City eating gefilte fish 'a la Veracruzana' too. Food keeps us connected."

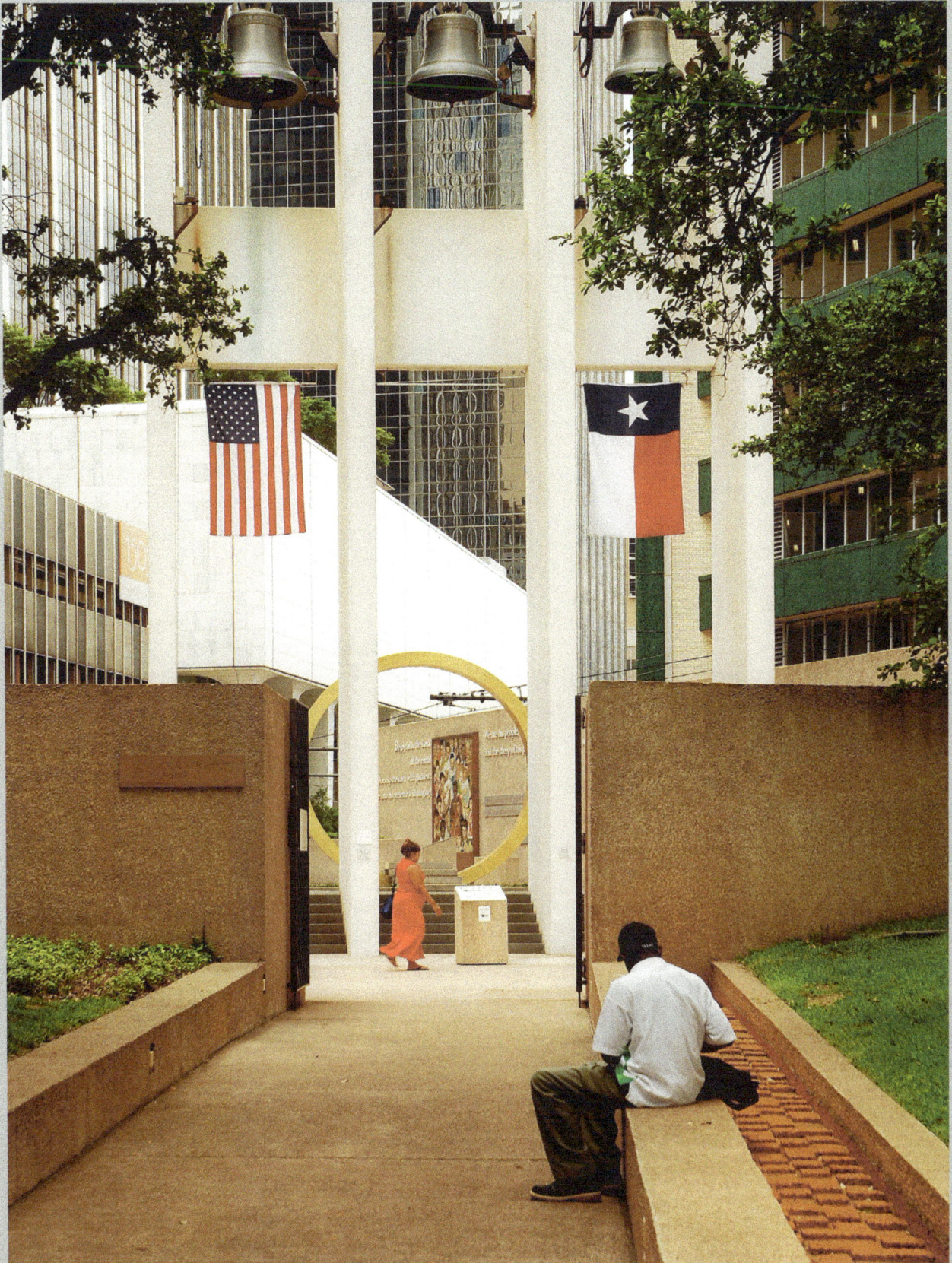

MEXICAN GEFILTE FISH

SERVES 4
PREPARATION: 50 MIN.

FISH DUMPLINGS
1 ¾ lb (800 g) red snapper
  or cod fillet, fresh or
  frozen, skin removed
2 medium onions
2 medium carrots
3 eggs
½ cup (60 g) matzo meal
Salt
Freshly ground white
  pepper

OLIVE-CAPER SAUCE
1 onion
2 tablespoons vegetable
  oil
2 cups (400 mL) fish stock
1, 15-oz can (400 g)
  chopped tomatoes
2 tablespoons ketchup
½ cup (100 g) manzanilla
  olives, stuffed with
  pimientos
3/4 cup (100 g) small,
  pickled peppers
2 tablespoons capers

TO SERVE
Toasted cornbread or
  fresh tortillas, to taste

FISH DUMPLINGS

1. Thoroughly clean, debone, and wash the fish fillet. Then thoroughly pat dry and coarsely chop. Peel and finely dice the onions. Peel and coarsely grate the carrots.
2. In a food processor, blend the fish into a coarse paste and place in a large bowl and set aside. Next, blend the carrots, onions, eggs, and matzo meal and add to the bowl with the fish paste. Stir together until uniform and season with salt and freshly ground white pepper. Cover and chill in the refrigerator.

OLIVE-CAPER SAUCE

1. Peel and finely dice the onion. In a large saucepan, heat the vegetable oil on medium-high heat and sweat the onion for about 5 minutes until translucent. Add the fish stock, tomatoes, and ketchup. Bring to a boil, reduce heat and simmer on low for 10 minutes until slightly thickened.
2. Meanwhile, with wet hands, form 12 oval, slightly flat dumplings from the cold fish mixture and place them side by side in the pan with the sauce. Cover the pan with a lid and gently cook for 15-20 minutes.
3. Cut half of the olives and half of the peppers into rings and add to the sauce along with 1 tablespoon of capers. Let simmer for another 5 minutes.
4. Arrange the remaining olives, peppers, and capers on a serving plate.

TO SERVE

Divide the fish balls among 4 plates and generously spoon some olive-caper sauce over the top. Serve with the accompanying plate of the remaining olives, peppers, and capers, and toasted slices of cornbread or fresh tortillas.

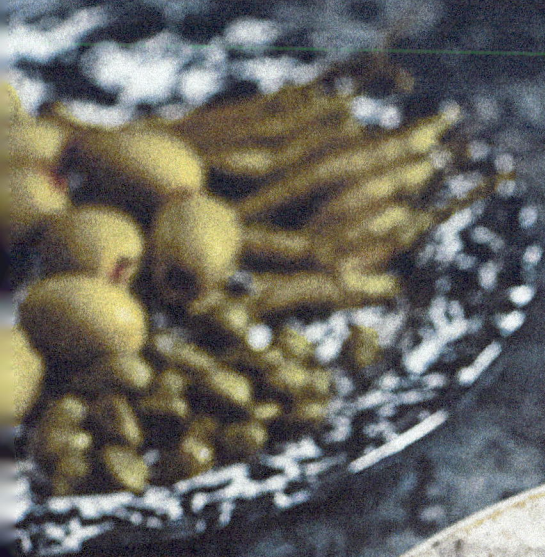

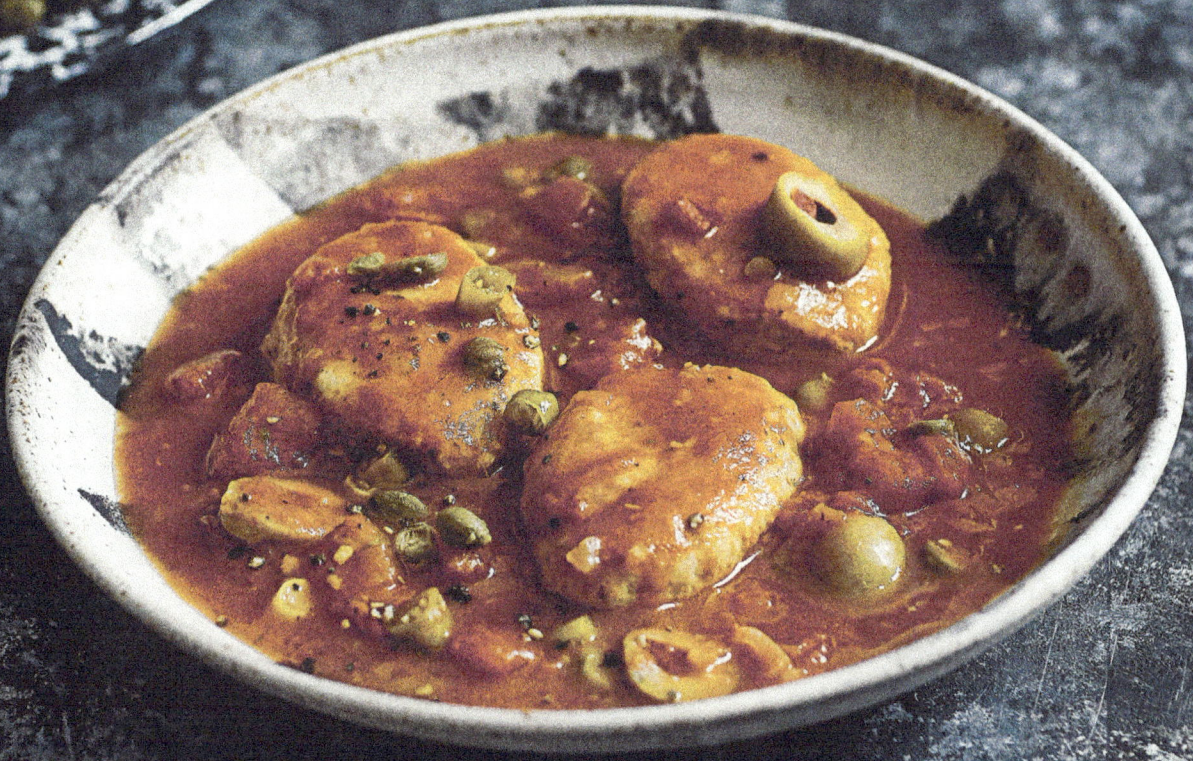

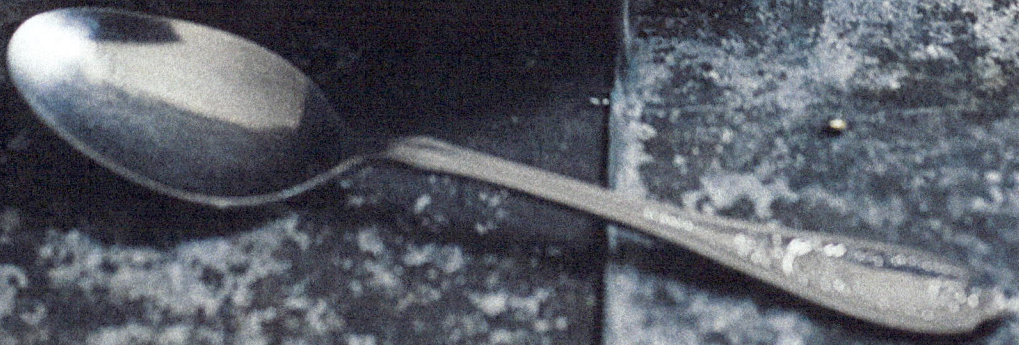

MATZO BALLS IN JALAPEÑO-MUSHROOM-SAUCE

SERVES 4
PREPARATION: 45 MIN.
SOAKING TIME: 1

MATZO BALLS
4 sprigs of flat-leaf
　parsley
2 cups (240 g) matzo meal
1 organic lemon
1 pinch of freshly grated
　nutmeg
2 eggs, beaten
2 tablespoons neutral
　vegetable oil
1 tablespoon water
Salt

SOUP
1 medium onion
1 clove of garlic
2 fresh jalapeño chilies
2 tablespoons neutral
　vegetable oil
3 cups (250 g) fresh white
　mushrooms
5 cups (1.2 L) chicken
　stock
Salt
Freshly ground black
　pepper

TO SERVE
4 fresh sprigs of parsley,
　to taste

MATZO BALLS
Place the matzo meal in a large bowl. Wash the lemon and zest a 1/4 of it and add to the bowl. Wash the parsley and pat dry. Pluck off the leaves and finely chop. Add parsley, freshly grated nutmeg, beaten eggs, vegetable oil, water, and 1 good pinch of salt and mix everything together. Cover and chill in the refrigerator for 1 hour.

MATZO SOUP
1. Finely dice the onion and garlic clove. Clean the jalapeño chili pepper, removing the seeds and membranes, and cut into fine rings. Heat the vegetable oil in a saucepan over medium-high heat. Add the onions, chilies, and garlic and sweat for 5 minutes until translucent.
2. Meanwhile, clean the mushrooms with a paper towel, remove brown ends and slice. Add the mushrooms to the pot, sauté for another 2 minutes. Cover the pot with a lid and let cook for another 6 minutes. Add the chicken stock and bring everything to a boil. Lower the temp and let simmer.
3. Remove the matzo-ball mixture from the refrigerator and form into 1-inch-thick balls with moistened hands until the mixture is used up. Add the matzo balls to the simmering soup and cook gently on the lowest setting for 20 minutes. Finally, season the soup with salt and freshly ground pepper.

TO SERVE
Divide the soup among 4 bowls, garnish each with 1 sprig of parsley, and serve hot.

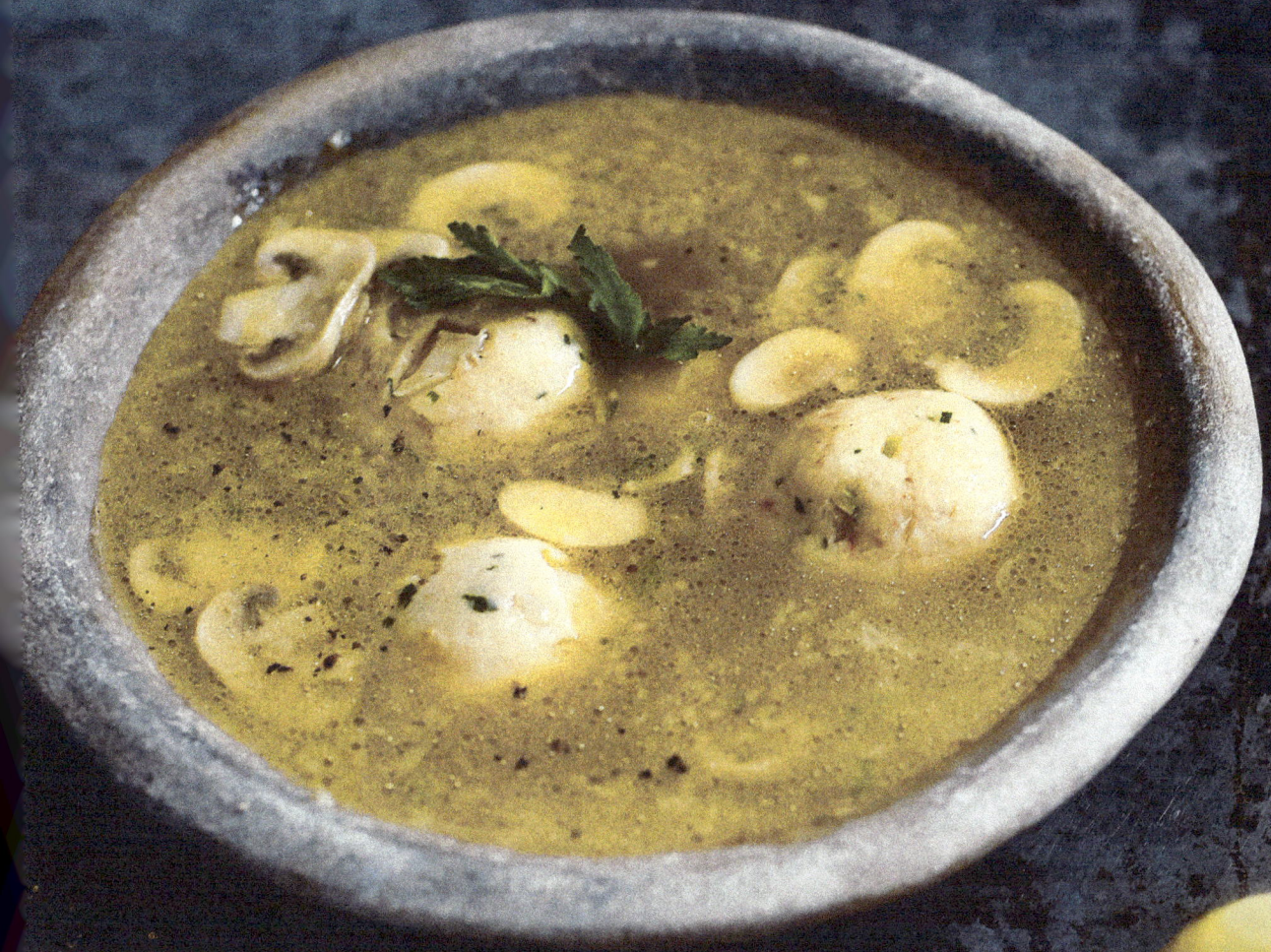

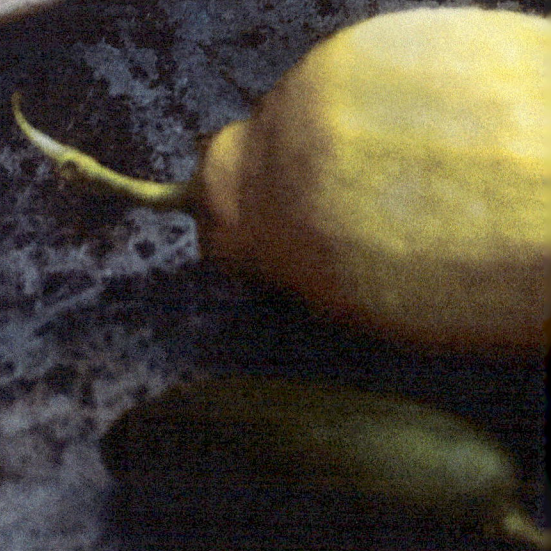

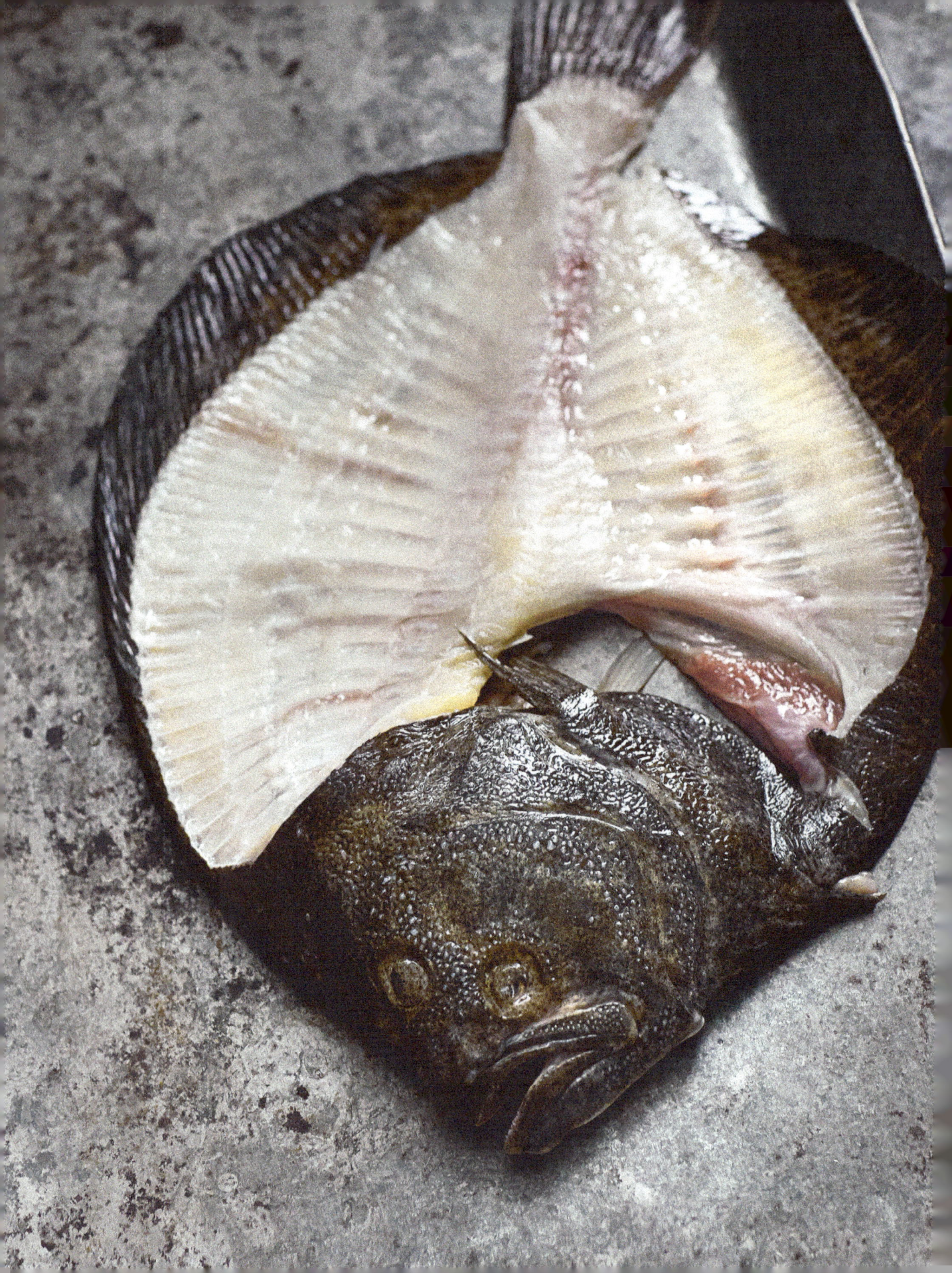

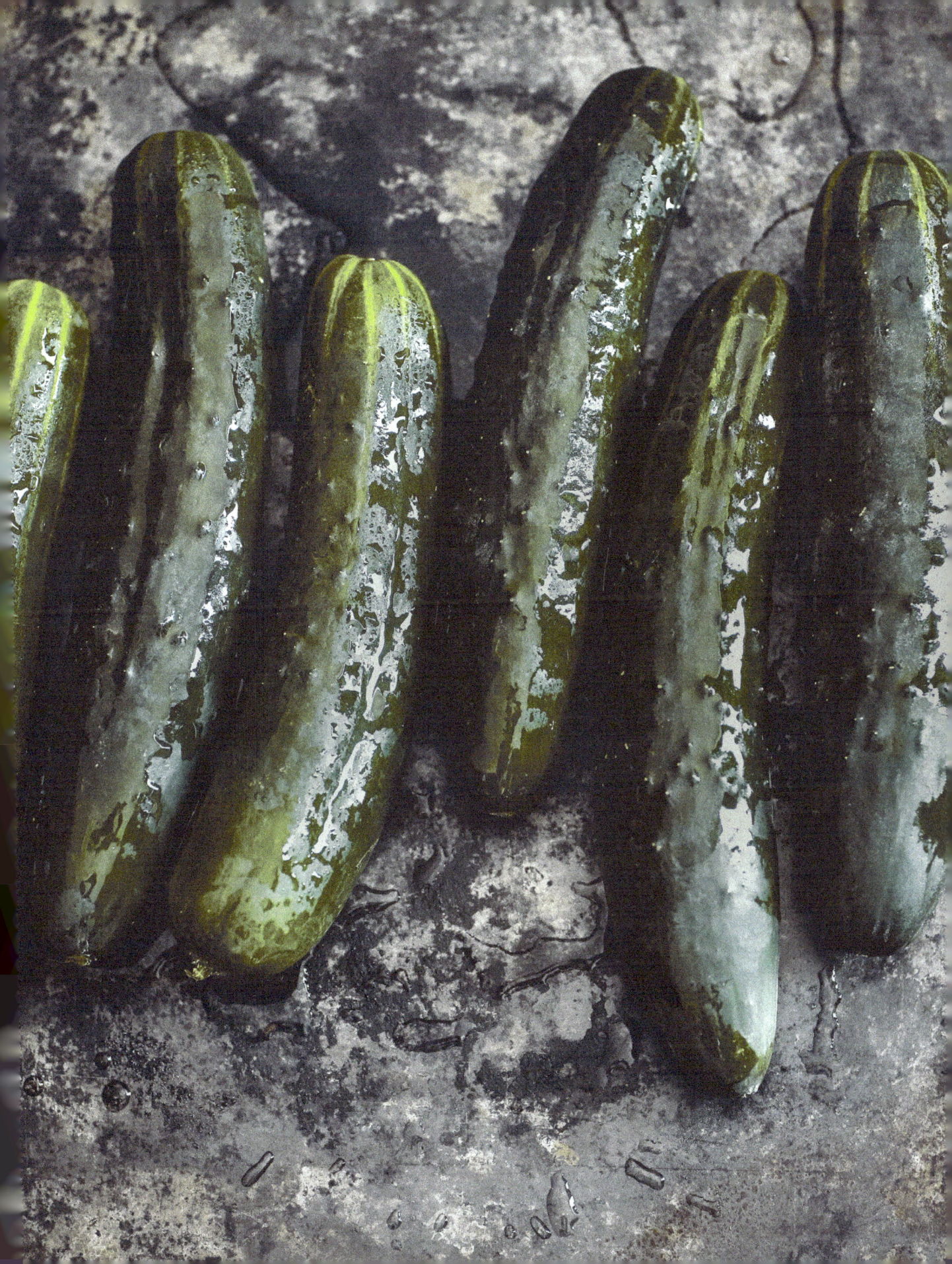

GLOSSARY

ASHKENASI
Eastern or Central European Jew

BABA GHANOUSH
Purée of eggplant and sesame paste

BORSCHT
Soup traditionally prepared with beets and very common in Eastern and Central Europe

BOTTARGA
salted mullet roe

CHALLAH
braided bread made from flour, yeast, eggs, and some fat; usually baked for Sabbat and Jewish holidays

CHOLENT
traditional Jewish stew, usually simmered for 12 hours or more, eaten at noon on Sabbat.

FALAFEL
fried balls of puréed beans or chickpeas, herbs, and spices

GEFILTE FISH
a cold fish dish especially popular among Ashkenazi Jews, eaten as an appetizer on Sabbat, holidays, and special occasions

GRIBENES
crispy fried chicken or duck skin

HARISSA
North African spice mixture

HOLISHKES
stuffed cabbage rolls

KASHA
buckwheat groats

KREPLACH
stuffed dumplings; traditional Ashkenazi-Jewish dish resembling Italian ravioli

KNISHES
small pies filled with such things as meat, potatoes, kasha, cheese, onions or vegetables; may be fried or baked

KOSHER

in Jewish religious tradition, ritually refers to "pure," "fit" or "suitable" foods, objects or actions; at the heart of a kosher lifestyle is the separation of meat and dairy products

KUBANEH

traditional Yemeni-Jewish yeast bread

KUGEL

traditional Ashkenazi-Jewish dish, which can resemble a casserole; there are sweet and savory variants; kugel can be a side dish or a dessert; it can be eaten hot or cold

LATKES

small, deep-fried potato pancakes, served as a side dish

LEKACH

honey cake

MATZO

unleavened bread; thin loaf of bread eaten by religious and traditional Jews during Passover; made from water and one of the five grains: wheat, rye, barley, oats or spelt

MATZO FLOUR

flour made from crushed matzo; replaces grain flour during the Passover period and is particularly characteristic of Ashkenazi Passover cuisine; also used throughout the year in the preparation of gefilte fish, matzo balls, cakes, egg cakes, and other dishes, and breadcrumbs

MATZO-BREI

an Ashkenasi dish often eaten as breakfast during Passover

PARVE

parve is the term used to describe foods that do not contain milk or meat; these include eggs, fruits, vegetables, grains, fish, and raw, unprocessed juices; a typical Jewish parve dish is gefilte fish

PETCHAH

Calves' foot jelly

RUGELACH

crescent-shaped pastries filled with such things as poppy seeds, cinnamon, chocolate, walnuts, or jam

SEMOLINA

fine wheat semolina

SEPHARDI

a Spanish-Portuguese or North African Jew

TAHINI

sesame paste

TARAMA

fish roe cream

TSIMMES

carrots cut into small cubes or slices, cooked on a low flame or in the oven and seasoned with honey and spices such as nutmeg or cinnamon, giving them a sweet and spicy flavor

USZKA

are small, filled dumplings whose shape resembles ears; typical fillings include sauerkraut, mushrooms, and meat. They are usually served as an accompaniment to clear soups or broths, like chicken soup

ZA'ATAR

African spice mixture

ZEITIM

olives

ZHUG

Yemeni spicy salsa

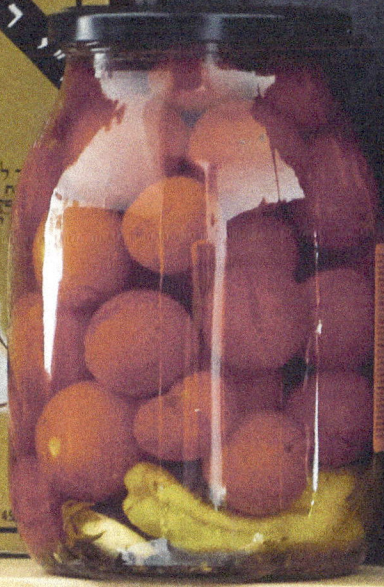

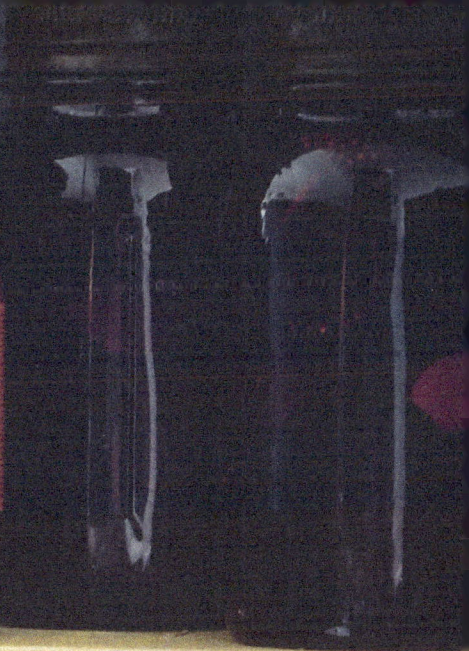

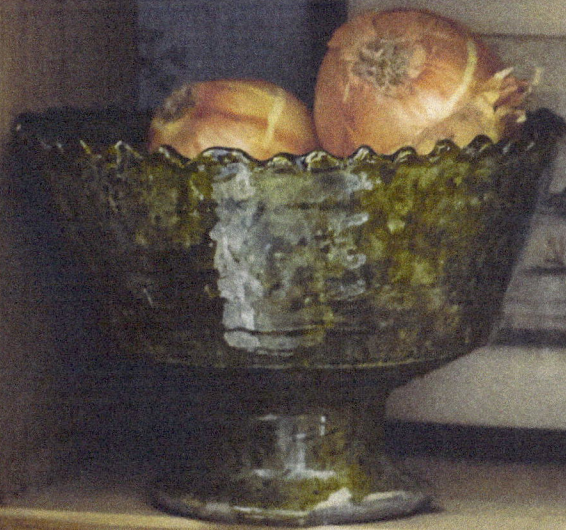

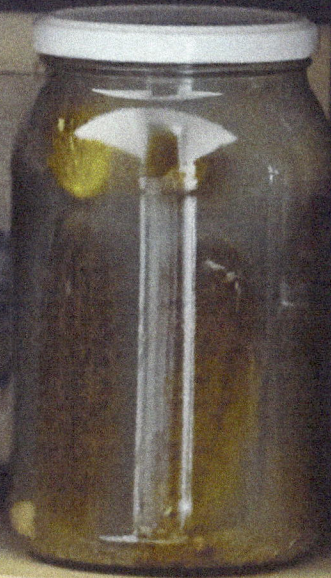

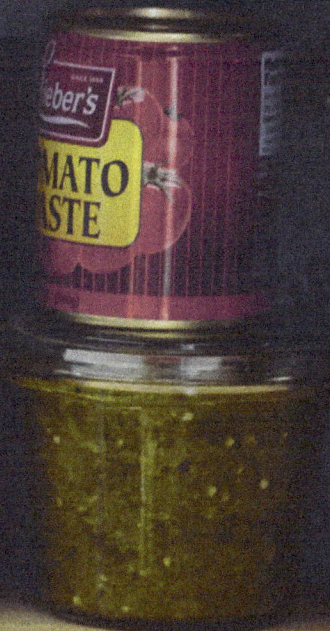

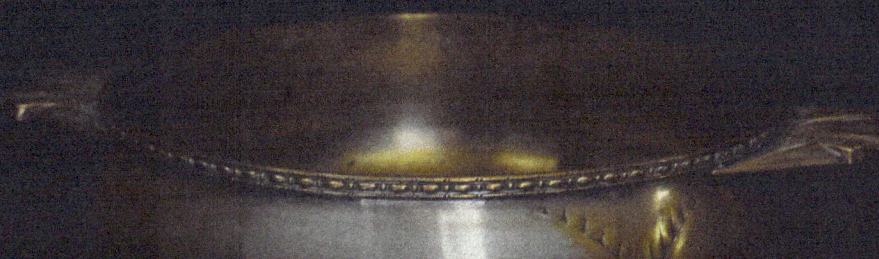

ADDRESSES

James & David Adinast
  Stanley Diamond
  Ottostraße 16–18
  60329 Frankfurt am Main
  www.stanleydiamond.com

  Chez Ima
  Niddastraße 58
  60329 Frankfurt am Main
  www.imaworld.de/restaurants/chezima.php

  Maxie Eisen
  Münchener Straße 18
  60329 Frankfurt am Main
  www.maxieeisen.com

Liz Alpern & Jeffrey Yoskowitz
  The Gefilteria – New York
  www.gefilteria.com

Arielle Artsztein
  Arielle's MACARONS Berlin
  Schillerstrasse 93
  10625 Berlin
  www.arielles-macarons.de

Avi Avital
  www.aviavital.com

Matan Choufan
  www.matanchoufan.com

Yossi Elad
  The Palomar Restaurant – London
  www.thepalomar.co.uk

Patricia Jinich
  www.patijinich.com

Jacob Kenedy
  Bocca di Lupo – London
  www.boccadilupo.com

  Gelupo – London
  www.gelupo.com

  Plaquemine Lock – London
  www.plaqlock.com

Leah Koenig
  www.leahkoenig.com

Anne Kornblut
    www.annekornblut.com

Sonja Lahnstein-Kandel
    www.step21.de

Laurel Kratochvila
    Fine Bagels Berlin
    Warschauerstraße 74,
    10243 Berlin
    www.finebagels.com

Kasia Leonardi
    www.jcckrakow.org/en

Itay Novik
    www.foodelements.net

Uri Scheft
    Breads Bakery – New York
    www.breadsbakery.com

Adeena Sussman
    www.adeenasussman.com

Molly Yeh
    www.mynameisyeh.com

Haya Molcho neni
    Naschmarkt 510
    1060 Wien
    www. neni.at/restaurants/naschmarkt/

    Höhe Obere Donaustraße 65
    1020 Wien
    www.neni.at/restaurants/tel-aviv-beach-bar/

    Budapester Straße 40
    10787 Berlin
    www.neniberlin.de

    Osakaallee 12 / Eingang Überseeboulevard
    20457 Hamburg
    www.nenihamburg.de

    Bahnhofplatz 1
    80335 München
    www.nenimuenchen.de

    Langstrasse 150
    8004 Zürich
    www.neni.ch

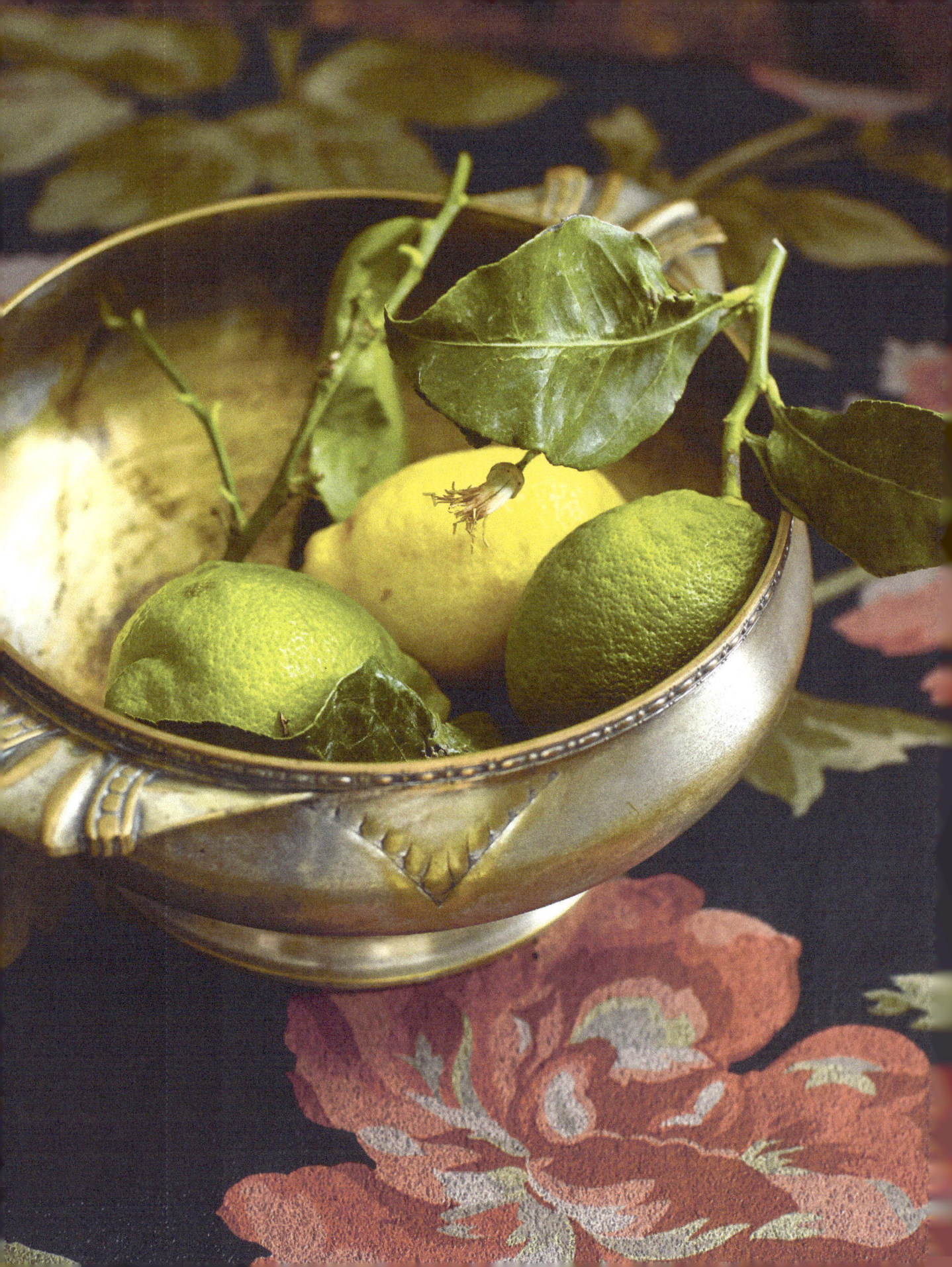

ACKNOWLEDGEMENTS

First and foremost, I would like to thank all the people who trusted me with their stories. At turns emotional, at turns humorous, but always enlightening and inspiring conversations have accompanied the creation of this book. I have learned an incredible amount from all the contributors. A common thread running through the conversations is the importance of listening to each other and of being together. At the end of the day, we're all just people trying to get through life as best we can and in between trying to do something good for our loved ones by preparing a good meal.

Special thanks go to Sonya Mayer from Christian Verlag. If Sonya had not found me in the far reaches of the internet, I wouldn't have had the pleasure of writing this book. I also have Maria Grossmann, who first conceived the idea for such a cookbook, and Monika Schuerle, with whom she took the amazing photos. The fact that the book has become such an incredibly beautiful object, which I will sleep with under my pillow every night, is entirely because of these two talented photographers.

Thanks also to Lukas Grossmann: co-author, chef, and food stylist extraordinaire. I can't imagine a better co-author.

Sarah Liewehr and Juliane Reichert, who spent over one year calmly listening to my complaints about writer's block and headaches and stress, and offered me lots of reassurance, encouraging me to continue. Claus Preisinger, the winemaker, and maker of Puszta Libre! Wine, which I drank by the liter while writing this book. Well chilled, it has always gotten the writer's juices flowing.

Ina Schulze, who read through and corrected my texts with an angelic calm and for whom I will be grateful all my life. Lastly, but very far from least, this book is dedicated to my father, Michael Fleischhacker. I have him to thank for so many things: for making me sandwiches for my school lunch and accompanying me to the train at 6:30 in the morning, every day until I was 18; for sending me to Jewish religious instruction for six years (even though I always complained, he wouldn't relent); for letting me come back to Judaism on my own, without ever pressuring me; and for the 110 percent support and love I have received over the past 30 years. Without him, nothing in my life would have been possible. Thank you, Dad.

AUTHORS

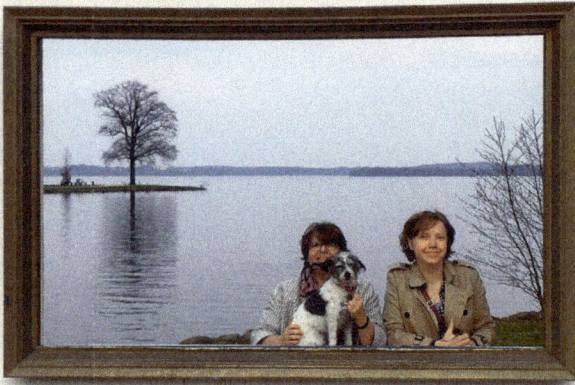
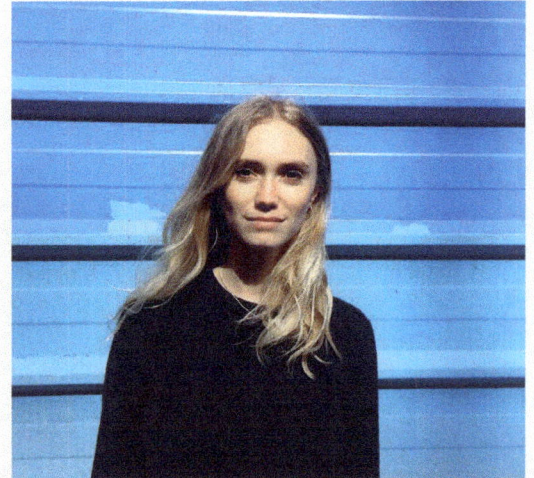
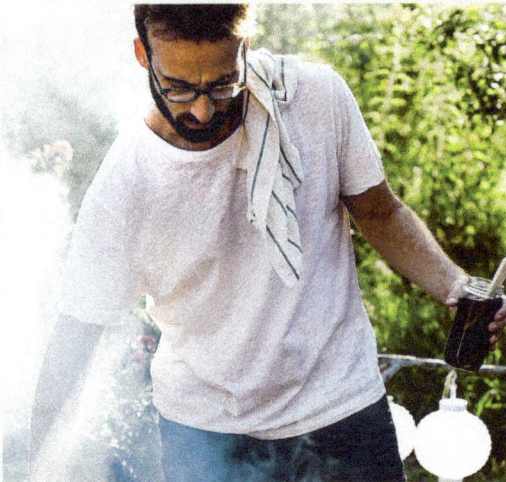
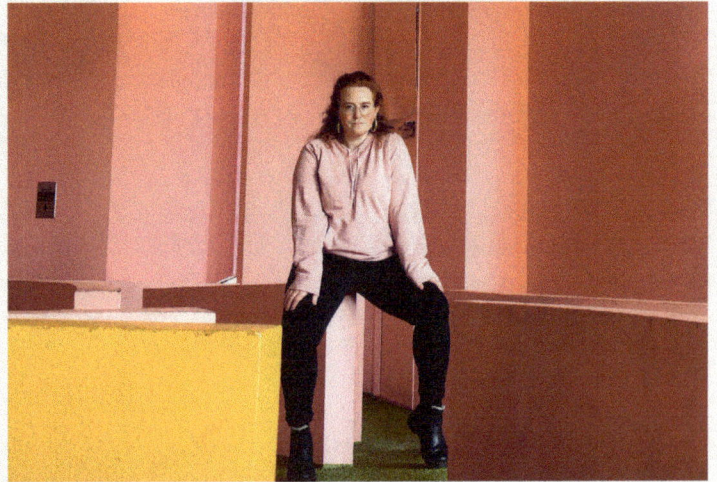

Clockwise from top left: Monika Schuerle and Maria Grossmann, Emily Schofield, Liv Fleischhacker, Lukas Grossmann

The idea for this book came to Maria Grossmann during a visit to Krakow. The fate of the Jews during the National Socialist era is particularly evident there, which led her to look more intensively into Jewish history. She asked herself what culinary memories the Jews who had emigrated from Europe had taken with them to their new homelands. And she also wondered how their descendants dealt with this heritage. Ultimately, Jewish cuisine cannot be reduced to a common denominator; it is a mixture of the old, new, and of different cultures in which the Jewish diaspora has settled. That's what makes Jewish cuisine so unique, exciting, and delicious.

MARIA GROSSMANN
& MONIKA SCHUERLE

The photo team Maria Grossmann and Monika Schuerle has been working together for years on topics related to food, still life, and interiors in Hamburg and Berlin. After Maria and Monika finished their education at the Lette Verein, Berlin, they took different paths. Monika stayed in Berlin and worked as a reportage and portrait photographer. Maria went to Hamburg and devoted herself to still life, interior, and food photography and worked with a lot of different photographers as a stylist. It was only years later that Monika and Maria began to start working on projects together, with food photography becoming the focus of their collaboration. The distribution of labor between them is fluid. Their clients include well-known publishing houses, agencies, and editorial offices at home and abroad.

LIV FLEISCHHACKER

Liv Fleischhacker is a native of Berlin and has been writing about food and drink culture since 2014. Having grown up between Berlin and Los Angeles, she is bilingual and writes in German and English. She is particularly familiar with the German capital's bars and founded Berlin's first Jewish Food Week, "Nosh Berlin," in early 2017. For *Mazel Tov!* she conducted the interviews and wrote the portraits.

LUKAS GROSSMANN

After completing his training as a chef in Hamburg, Lukas Grossmann completed various internships, including at the three-star Aqua restaurant in Wolfsburg and in the test kitchen of the German monthly magazine, Essen & Trinken. Among his other culinary experiences, he spent time working on a farm in Namibia and at the trendy food hall, Markthalle 9 in Berlin, where he now also lives. His numerous long visits to Japan, Southeast Asia, and Australia, have greatly expanded his culinary knowledge, which he now uses as a freelance chef, recipe author, and food stylist. He wrote the recipes for *Mazel Tov!*

EMILY SCHOFIELD

Emily Schofield studied graphic design at Central Saint Martin's College of Art and Design in London. After graduation, she did internships and freelance work at the design studios Praline in London and Spassky Fischer in Paris. Meanwhile, the German-English native of Hamburg works as a freelancer on various commissions for international artists, designers, publishers, and cultural institutions. She oversaw the design for *Mazel Tov!*

Index
—Recipes

PICTURE CREDITS

All of the photos in this book come from Grossmann and Schuerle,
with the exception of the following:

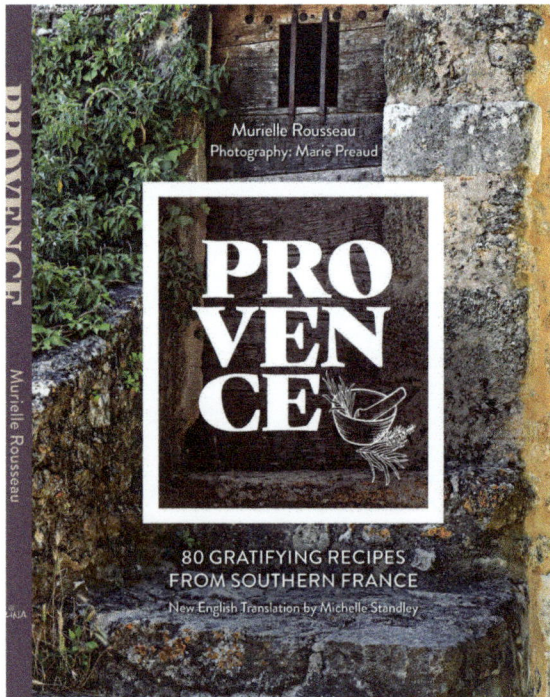

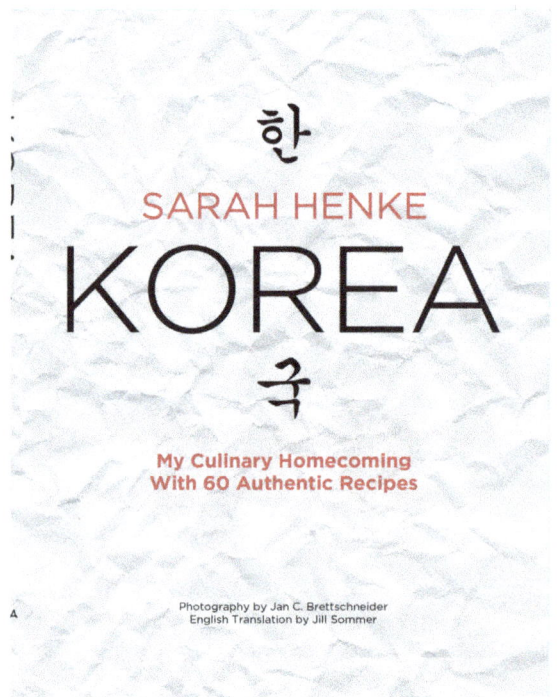

OTHER TITLES YOU MAY ENJOY
from

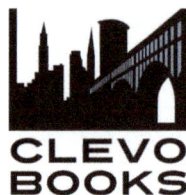

an imprint of

CLEVO BOOKS

www.ingramcontent.com/pod-product-compliance
Ingram Content Group UK Ltd.
Pitfield, Milton Keynes, MK11 3LW, UK
UKHW052307130725
460650UK00004B/22

9 780997 305